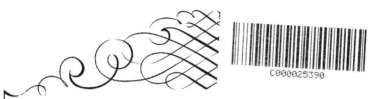
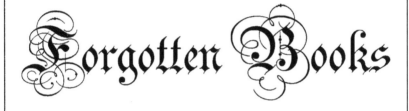
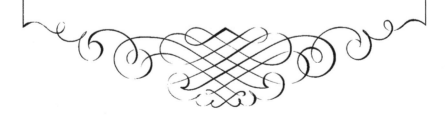

ISBN 978-0-260-17426-0
PIBN 11018141

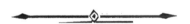

English
Français
Deutsche
Italiano
Español
Português

www.forgottenbooks.com

Mythology Photography **Fiction**
Fishing Christianity **Art** Cooking
Essays Buddhism Freemasonry
Medicine **Biology** Music **Ancient**
Egypt Evolution Carpentry Physics
Dance Geology **Mathematics** Fitness
Shakespeare **Folklore** Yoga Marketing
Confidence Immortality Biographies
Poetry **Psychology** Witchcraft
Electronics Chemistry History **Law**
Accounting **Philosophy** Anthropology
Alchemy Drama Quantum Mechanics
Atheism Sexual Health **Ancient History**
Entrepreneurship Languages Sport
Paleontology Needlework Islam
Metaphysics Investment Archaeology
Parenting Statistics Criminology
Motivational

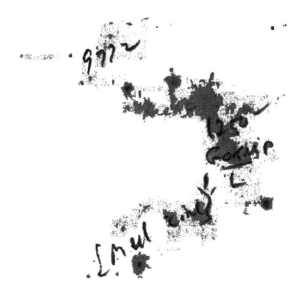

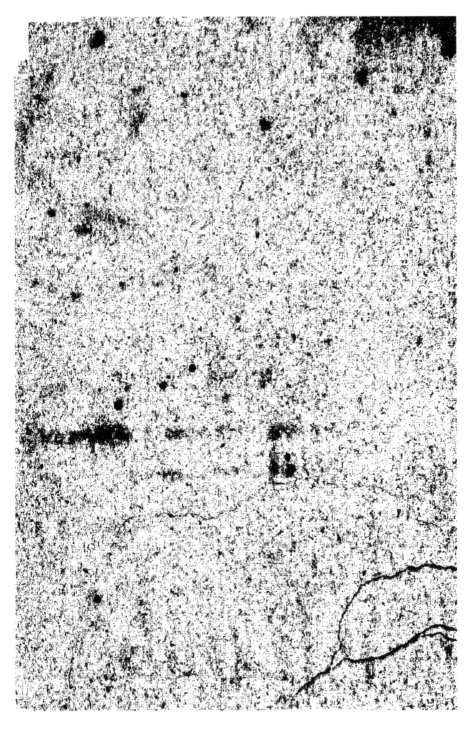

THE

INDIAN GUIDE TO HEALTH,

OR

VALUABLE

VEGETABLE MEDICAL PRESCRIPTIONS

FOR THE

USE OF FAMILIES,

OR

YOUNG PRACTITIONERS.

~~~~~~~~~~~~~~~~~~~~

PUBLISHED BY J. H, STEVENS & J. C. CORY,
ST. LOUIS, MISSOURI,

~~~~~~~~~~~~~~~~~~~~

J. ROSSER & BROTHER, PRINTERS,
LAFAYETTE, IND.
1845.

PRICE, $5,00

THE

INDIAN GUIDE TO HEALTH,

OR

VEGETABLE MEDICAL PRESCRIPTION,

FOR THE

USE OF FAMIL

YOUNG PRACTITIONERS.

INTRODUCTION.

IN all ages of the world the Science of Medicine has engaged the particular attention of the most learned of every nation; and of late years, the time and talents of a few eminent individuals have been employed in communicating to their fellow men, desertation upon DOMESTIC MEDICINE; for which, they have been censured by a majority of the medical faculty, who, with the most audacious effronty, assert that, by so doing, "Every man is made his own physician;" and the consequent result is, that a majority of these who pretend that they have made themselves acquainted with all diseases, and their proper remedies, have to resort to some other occupation to gain a livelihood, and the Science is thereby injured.

Works heretofore published on the subject of Domestic Medicine, though good in many respects, have greatly failed in a general usefulness, and for the reason that they are written in a style not familiar to the common ear. Technicle names have been given to almost all diseases and also their appropriate remedies, which has in a degree rendered them useless to seven-eights of the citizens of this country. To remedy which evil, the author in this work, has endeavored to treat, in the most clear and concise manner all diseases to which the human body is subject—to give them common names—to point out their surest symptoms—original causes, and apporpriate remedies, prepared by distillation, extracts, &c., &c., from the superabundant Garden of Nature.

The greater part of the author's information in the science of medicine, he obtained from Dr. RICHARD CARTER of Shelby County, Kentucky, who is commonly called the "INDIAN DOCTOR;" on whom all the powers of ratiocination in possession of the faculty were expended without effect. To which he has added six years experience in almost unlimited practice in all the diseases of this climate, and during which time, in almost a thousand instances, he has seen his medicine have the most happy effects in the cure of disorders, after the skill of the heretofore popular faculty, had been baffled in the administration of their calomel, and the patients given over by them to die.

In a country like this, where people are so subject to violent attacks of disease, and where the chances to obtain medical aid in such, are so uncertain, a work of this description must be of great utility ; in fact, every family should be in possession of one ; not because it would be found useful in extreme cases, but because in the most slight attacks, it would be found a ready and sure guide—a guide by which a person of but ordinary abilities, can administer medicine without fear of injuring the patient.

The reader will find in the latter part of this work, a METERIA MEDICA, which points out the "simples" wherewith the divine Creator has, in His wisdom, planted our "gardens, fields and woods," for the healing of our infirmities.

In the conclusion there is a general index, by a refference to which the reader can in a moment, point to any particular disease and its remedy.

A great deal of the future health of man, depends on his organization and rise in the world. A child born of healthy parents ; and being exposed to the different elements at or near its birth, that is of cold water or air, with other changes, such children generally bring into the world a system by nature formed to resist the cause of disease. The treatment of children among us Indians tends to secure this firmness of constitution, that becomes in some degree hereditary. To harden them against the inclemency of the weather we plunge our pappooses frequently under water, winter and summer and to preserve their shape, we tie them to a board for several months our children are frequently part naked and either bare footed or wear a kind of thin mockasin which is but little defence against water or cold, our wigwams part open and even some times without wigwams and the top of our heads are all ways open to the snow or rain, in this way our constitutions are prepared to stand the inclemency of the weather. In the time of plenty and in war and more especially in victory ; we rise in victorious exercise and strike a lance ; having little bells or heeds tied to our ancles and instruments in our hands to make a noise, and we parade around the fire in winter ; and in summer around other objects over which we make motions as though we would tommahawk or scalp each other, and try our activity to see how near we can strike at another's head and still miss it, and every few rounds we always raise a shout and thus set our blood in a high state of circulation, our squaws always stand near one place in their dance and shuffle their feet having a number of deers hoofs and the like fastened near the bottom of their garments while they make a low and rather a coarse noise. Our squaws does the principal part of the hard work, this gives a firmness to their bodies and strength to their constitution, their menses seldom begin to flow before they are eighteen years of age and cease before they are forty; and they seldom marry till they are above twenty-five. During pregnancy our women are excused from the more laborious parts of their labor., Nature is their only midwife. Each woman is delivered in a private wigwam without so much as one of her own sex to attend her, and after washing herself in cold water, she returns in a few days to her own camp.

POCAHONTUS NONOQUET.

TINEA, or SCALLED HEAD.

This disease consists in a chronic inflamation of the skin of the head, productive of a secretion of matter peculiar in its nature, and capable of propagating the complaint, if applied to the healthy scalp of a subject. At first, the eruption is confined, probably only to a small portion of the head; but by degrees its acrimony is extended to the neighboring parts, and at length the whole of the scalp is eroded, and best with a scabby eruption. Dr. Willan has substituted the term porigo for that of tinea, asbeing less objectionable, and considers this genus as consisting of several variations. Children are principally affected with it particularly those of the poor; hence it evidently arises from uncleanliness, from the want of a due proportion of wholesome nutritive food and possibly from bad nursing. At any rate, these will very much aggravate the disease. In many instances, it is propagated by contagation, either by using a comb imbued with the matter from the head of a person laboring under it, or by putting on his hat or cap.— When proper means are adopted, the disease seldom proves of difficult cure. The hair should be shaven off the head, and then covered with an ointment made of dog wood berries, and the flowers of mulberry, stewed together in sweet oil or hogs lard, this should be used every night and morning, the head should be frequently washed in castile soap and new milk it also may be washed at times in copperas water, if the gland of the neck should become swelled, a small blister should be drawn on the back of the neck, and be kept a running a few days, by pursuing this course there is no difficulty of performing a cure.

INCUBUS, OR NIGHT-MARE.

This is evidently a nervous affection, and comes on during sleep, with a sense of considerable weight and suppression at the chest, the person making many efforts to speak and move without effect, until, after many deep groans and much mourning, he at length awakes greatly frightened, and feels a considerable palpitation at the heart, with tremors, anxiety, and lasitude. The causes which give rise to this complaint, are chiefly anxiety, grief, despondency, and intense thought ; but it is sometimes occasioned by making use of food of a hard indigestible nature for supper. In most cases it may, however, be considered as arising from the impression of dreams, or a distemperature of thought, and therefore is not attended with any great danger. A spasmodic constriction of the diaphragm and muscles of the chest, is by manyr assigned as the proximate cause of incubus. Those who lead an inactive sedentary life, and are of a lax fibre, are most predisposed to its attacks. The remedies. The first thing necessary is to cleanse the blood ; that is to get a handful of the bark of the root of yellow poplar, the same as dogwood bark, the north side ; the same of wild cherrytree bark, the same of yellow sarsaparilla root, and the same of the roots of running brier, put these in a copper kettle and put a quart of water to every handful, and boil it slowly away to two quarts, then add a pint of whiskey, take a table spoonful two or three times a day ; let your diet be chickens, squirrels beef, mutton, and broths, not too highly seasoned. Or get a handful of wild cherrytree bark, the same of running brier roots, the same of burdock roots, the same of sassafras bark, the same of white ash tops, add a quart of water to every handful, boil it half away ; drink this for your constant drink, and take fifteen drops of the essence of peppermint on going to bed.

ANASARCA, OR DROPSY IN THE CELLULAR MEMBRANCE.

This species of dropsy shows itself at first with a swelling of the feet and ancles, towards evening, which for a time disappears in the morning. The tumefaction is soft and easy dented, and when pressed upon with the finger, retains its mark for some time, the skin becoming much paler than usual. By degrees the swelling ascends upwards and occupies the thighs and trunk of the body, and at last even the face and eyelids appear full and bloated. When it has become pretty general, the viscera are affected in a similar way; the cellular membrance of the lungs partakes the affection, the breathing then becomes difficult, and is accompanied by cough, and the expectoration of a watery fluid; the urine is small in quantity, and deposits a reddish sediment; sometimes, however, it is of a pale whey color, and more copious; the belly is costive the perspiration much obstructed, the countenance yellow and a considerable degree of thirst, with amaciation of the whole body prevails. To these symptoms succeed torpor, heaviness, and a slow fever. In some cases the water oozes out through the pores of the cuticle; in others, being too gross to pass by these, it raises the cuticle in small blisters and sometimes the skin, not allowing the water to escape through it, is compressed and hardened, and is at the same time so much discharged, as to give the tumor a considerable degree of firmness. The disease is always to be regarded as admitting more readily of a cure, when it arises from topical weakness or general debility, than when it has been occasioned by viserial obstruction; likewise when recent, than when it has been of a very long continuance. The skin becoming somewhat moist, with a diminution of thirst, and an increase in the flow of urine, are to be regarded as very favorable symptoms. In some few cases, nature makes powerful efforts of her own accord and the disease goes off by a spontaneous

crisis, either by a vomiting, purging or an unusual discharge of urine; but this does not often happen. Con-
comitant organic disease, great emaciation, erysipela-
tous inflamation, much drowsiness, petechiae and ecy-
mosis, hemorrhage, febrile heat, great thirst. and a quick
small pulse, are very unfavorable symptoms, In dropsical cases we should always carefully investigate whether the disease is an original one, or prevails as a symptom of some other; for by removing the cause, we
shall often be able to perform a cure. . For instance, it
it has arisen as the consequence of intemperance, a free
use of spirituous liquors, exposure to a moist atmosphere, or the having had resource to large evacuations,
particularly by bleeding, these ought carefully to be
avoided in future; or if it has proceeded from long-
continued intermittents, obstructions in the abdominia
or thoracie viscera, and the like, these should be obviated, by the mildest of means, in the first place it is necessary, that a general flow of blood should be produced through the extremities, as it is frequently the case
that the blood is confined to the breast and head, in order to produce this circulation of blood, and to keep
down inflamation, you will get, one peck of green plantain, the same of liverwort, the same of winter green,
the same of burdock, the same of the blossoms of philadelphia flea-bane, the same of polk-berries, the same
of dog-wood berries, you will put these ingredients together in a large kettle or still, boil them in fifteen gallons of water down to three gallons, then strain the
liquid from the vegetables, add to the liquid two pounds
of Epsom-salts, one pint of the tincture of gumguiacum,
one quart of hard cider, half an ounce of the rust of
iron, the same of salamoniac, you will then boil this
down to one gallon, it is then fit for use; the patient
may take from a tea spoonful to a table spoonful, three
times a day, refraining from all strong diet, this medicine will have the tendency of assuaging the swelling
in a short time, and acts very powerfully upon the urine.

So soon as the swelling begins to subside, get a handful of the inside bark of dog wood, the same of the inside bark of yellow poplar, the same of featherfew, the
same of Indian turnip, the same of horsemint, these articles are to be boiled in two gallons of cider or weak
vinegar or water, down to half a gallon, take it out and
strain it, to this you will add, four ounces of loaf sugar,
twenty grains of refined nitre, of this preparation the
patient should use one table spoonful every night and
morning, if there should be any soreness in the bowels
while using of this medicine, a small portion of paragoric may be mixed with each dose, if the bowels are
costive the patient should use the cream of tartar, senna, manna, castor oil, &c. The body of the patient
should be rubed all over with a piece of warm flannel
every night and morning, wine and water should be
frequently used, a few drops of elixir vitriol may be taken in a little weak tody, once or twice a day, beware
of getting cold, or fatigue, I have laid down the symptoms of this disease in the first place, in the second
place my mode of treatment, so that the citizens of
the country may know the complaint and the remedies
necessary to be used in such cases, though the prescriptions are simple yet powerful and effectual when properly administered.

ASCITES, OR DROPSY IN THE BELLY.

This disease is marked by a tense swelling of the abdomen, accompanied by an evident fluctuation. The
water is usually collected in the sac of the peritonaeum,
or general cavity of the abdomen; but sometimes it is
found entirely without the peritonaeum, and between
this and the abdominal muscles. Collections of water
in so meinstances, begin by sacs formed upon and connected with one or other of the visera, as happens frequently in the ovarea of women. These form that dis-

ease which has been termed encysted dropsy. Hyda-
tids have been supposed to give rise to them. "In addition to the causes which have been enumerated as
productive of anasarca, certain local affections, as diseases of the viscera of the abdomen; scirrhosities of
the liver, spleen, or pancreas; enlargement of the me-
sentiric glands, local injury, &c. do sometimes occasion
ascites.   Ascites is often preceded by loss of appetite,
sluggishness, inactivity, dryness of the skin, oppression
of the chest, diminution of the natural discharges of
urine, and costiveness.   Shortly after the appearance
of these symptoms, a protuberance is perceived in the
hypogastrium, which extends gradually and keeps increasing, until the whole abdomen becomes at length
uniformly swelled and tense.   The distention and sense
of weight, although considerable, vary somewhat according to the posture of the body, the weight being
felt the most in that side on which the patient lies,
while at the same time the distention becomes somewhat less on the opposite one.   In general the patient
may be sensible of the fluctuation of the water, by applying his left hand on one side of the abdomen, and
then striking on the other with his right.   In some
cases it will be obvious to the ear.   As the collection
of water becomes more considerable, the difficulty of
breathing is much increased, the countenance exhibits
a pale or bloated appearance, and immoderate thirst
arises, the skin is dry and parched, and the urine is very scanty, thick, and high-colored, and deposits a lateritious sediment.   In the general dropsy, the urine, co-
agueates like the diluted serum of the blood, whilst in
that which proceeds from unsound viscera, it is usually
high colored, scanty and on cooling deposits a pink
colored sediment.   With respect to the pulse it is variable, being sometimes considerably quickened, and at
other times slower than natural.   Although ascites is
sometimes accompanied by fever, still it is frequently
absent.   It has, however, been observed, that during

ascites, the derangement in the general system is greater than in other respects of dropsy. In the treatment
of ascites, we are to attend to the two following indi-
cations, first, to evacuate the accumulated, fluid: second
and to prevent any fresh collection to answer the first
of these intentions, it is necessary to have recourse to
purgatives of the following kind, you will get half a
peck of the inside bark of white walnut, the same of
the inside bark of dogwood, the same of the roots of
elder, the same of alecampane, to these you will add
six gallons of water, and boil it down to half a gallon,
strain it in the usual way, to this you will add one pint
of molasses, of this preparation, the patient should
take one table spoonful three times per day, if in case
it should operate too powerful upon the bowels, the
quantity may be decreased, this medicine will have the
tendency of carrying off the water by the bowels and
urine after this course has been pursued five or six days,
you will stop this course, and take the following: take
four ouncee of jalap, the same of cream of tartar,
half ounce of pulverised columbo root, half an ounce
of pulverised squill root, of this you will take half a
table spoonful every night and morning, at the same
time use a tea of horsemint or parsley, this medicine
will have the effect of carrying off the water in the
same way of the other preparation above mentioned,
this course should be pursued until the water should be
measurably carried off, it is now necessary that the
regular digestive powers of the system, should be restored by mild tonics such as the following: the patient
should take from ten to thirty drops of the tincture of
quinine or the essence of orange, in a little water four
or five times a day, the patient should be frequently
bathed in strong salted water, immediately afterwards
should be wrapped up in warm flannel cloths. Should
there appear to be any fever, the sweet spirits of nitre
should be used from a tea spoonful to half a table spoonful, two or three times a day until the fever subsides

should the bowels become costive, rheubarb and peruvian bark, should be frequently used, by this course of
treatment, there is no difficulty of performing a cure
if taken in time.

SPRAINS.

, Accidents of this nature happen most frequently in
the wrists, knees and ancles; and are usually occasioned by a slip, or some sudden effort or violent exertion.
Sprains of the tendons and ligaments are usually productive of immediate painful and inflammatory swelling. In severe sprains there is often not only an increased action of the arteries in the inflamed part, but
there is likewise an instantaneous effusion from the
rupture of some of the small vessels. In general, we
may suppose the effusion to be of the serous kind, as
the skin is not altered in colour for some time after the
accident; but it sometimes happens that the tumid parts
are either of a deep red or leaden colour from the very
first, owing to blood being extravasated from the ruptured vessels. In the treatment of sprains, two circumstances are principally to be attended to: the first,
to prevent, by all possible means, the swelling from ar-
riving at any considerable magnitude; the second, to
employ those remedies which are known to be powerful in removing inflammation. To answer the first of
these intentions, restringent applications, such as vinegar, ardent spirits, the lees of red wine may be made
use of. By immersing the injured part in any of these
immediately on receiving the injury, the effusion will be
rendered much less than it otherwise would be and perhaps be altogether prevented. Plunging the sprained
limb into the coldest water that can be procured as soon
after the accident as possible, is often attended with the
basteffect. and may be advised as the first step, till one

or other of the articles just mentioned can be procured. To answer the second intention of removing inflamma- tion, we may have resource to blood letting, f the pain and inflamation does not subside readily, we should have recourse to cooling medicines such as, salts, &c. And such as are generally used in cases of inflammation. Where a weakness remains in consequence of a sprain, a preparation of turpentine, camphor, sweet oil, or hogs lard, of equal quantities of each, an ointment made of the same. The part should be well rubbed every night and morning warmed by the fire, at the same time wearing flannel round the affected parts. This treatment seldom fails of performing a cure.

ASTHMA.

This disease is a spasmodic affection of the lungs, which comes on by paroxysms most generally at night, and is attended by a frequent, difficult, and short respi- ration, together with a wheezing noise, tightness across the chest, and a cough, all of which symptoms are much increased when the patient is in a horizontal po- sition. Asthma rarely appears before the age of puber- ty, and seems to attack men more frequently than women, particularly those of a full habit, in whom it never fails, by frequent repetition, to occasion some degree of emaciation. Dyspepsy always prevails, and appears to be a very prominent feature in the predispo- sition. Its attacks are most frequent during the heats of summer, and in winter when heavy fogs or sharp cold winds prevail. When the disease is attended with an accumulation and discharge of humors from the lungs, it is called the humid asthma, but when it is unaccom- panied by any expectoration, it is known by the name of the dry or spasmodic asthma. On the evening pre- ceding an attack of asthma the spirits are often much affected, and the person experiences a sense of fullness

about the stomach, with lassitude drowsiness, and a pain
in the head. On the approach of the succeeding evening he perceives a sense of tightness and stricture
across the breast, and a sense of straightness in the
lungs impeding respiration. The difficulty of breathing continuing to increase for some length of time,
both in aspiration and expiration, are performed slowly,
and with a wheezing noise; the speech becomes difficult and uneasy, a propensity to coughing succeeds,
and the patient can no longer remain in a horizontal
position, being as it were threatened with immediate
suffocation.

These symptoms usually continue till towards the
approach of morning, and then a remission commonly
takes place; the breathing becomes less laborious and
more full, and the person speaks and coughs with greater ease. If the cough is attended with an expectoria-
tion of mucus, he experiences much relief, and soon
falls asleep. In the management of this disease, it will
be well to bear in mind, that laxity of fibre, and morbid
sensibility and irritability are the predominant features
of the asthma. We should avoid all violent medicines.
As the asthma so frequently arises from a disordered
state of stomach and bowels, the employment of laxative medicines affords great relief, the purgatives may
be the tincture of rhubarb, or castor-oil, may be freely
used in all attacks, when there appears to be great difficulty in breathing, it will be necessary to use tartarized
antimony or a tincture of lobelia. In order to produce
a general expectoration from the lungs, and to restore
the digestive powers, the patient should take the following preparation: get half a bushel of angelico roots,
the same of spignard roots, the same of the inside bark
of yellow poplar, add those ingredients together, boil
them in six gallons of water to half a gallon, take out
the vegetables and strain it, to this add one pint of
French brandy, two pounds of white sugar, of this
take half a table spoonful three times per day, with

tea spoonful of sweet oil—the oxygen of squills should also be used at times, tonics, such as barks and quinine should also be used. I have had many cases of this kind though it is thought by the most of writers to be incurable, yet I have relieved many, and made them well, as they were previous to the attack.

Though my medicine is much condemned, and said to be nothing more than roots, herbs, and barks, yet many can tell the good effects it has had on them.— "Tho'" Indian medicine—as they are called, they have relieved the afflicted pain: of those patients who to me have came.

I feel in hopes that mankind will soon begin to discover, that in the garden of nature there are medicines for all diseases to which the human body afflicted.

THE THRUSH.

This is a very common complaint among young children. Its approach may be known and stopped by a few doses of the powders to wit: take of magnesia twenty grains, of rheubarb five grains, these must be powdered and mixed together and for a dose take down three to five grains every six hours. When this disease takes place, the tongue becomes in some degree swelled; its color and that of the throat, is purple; ulcers appear first on the throat, edges of the tongue, and at length over the whole mouth. These ulcers, are of a whitish color; sometimes they are quite distant, and in some instances run together. The time of its duration is uncertain. For the cure, let the mouth be carefully and gently washed several times in the day, with the following solution : To half a gill of water well sweetened with honey or molasses, add fifteen grains of borax, when disolved, it is ready for use, or if this is not

2

convenient, take sage tea, half a gill, sweetened as before, add to it from five to ten grains of the best almond
soap to be used as above ; or take a handful of brier
roots, the same of persimmon tree bark, the same of
privay, the same of white oak bark, the same of common cherry tree twiggs, and the same of sage ; boil
these articles all together well, and strain it, then add a
tea spoonful of alum, half a pint of honey, half a tea
spoonful of salt peter, and a little vinegar, and wash
the mouth twice or thrice a day this is a certain cure.

PESORA OR ITCH.

This complaint is evidently confined to the skin and
never affects the general system, however, great its irritation. The disease is evidently a very contagious one
and may be communicated by coming in contact with
the body of a person already affected or by wearing
the same clothes or by lying in the same bed linen that
he has done. But it is sometimes produced by unwholesome food, bad air, and neglect ot cleanliness, &c. A
good deal more might be said concerning its pathol-
ogy, but I presume it unnecessary as it is a disease with
which the most of persons are well acquainted. The
surest method of treatment is as follows :—Take a
handful of sourdock roots, the same of bark of dogwood root, the same of the bark of elder root, the same
of balsam, the same of the bark of sassafras roots, a
piece of poke root as large as a goose egg, all boiled
well together, then strained and stewed slowly down
to the consistency of syrup, then take it off, and stir half
cold, add two spoonfuls of tar to one pint of the dococ-
tion, one spoonful of salt petre, the same soft soap
the same of sulphur, the same of black pepper beat fine,
all this to be stewed well together, it may be rubbed
on the joints, or all over the body it necessary. This
is good to cure any itching humors.

THE TETTER WORM.

To cure this disease, get a good chance of white hickory bark, also the inside bark of black oak, boil these well together and strain it, then put it back in the vessel, add a little blue stone and copperas, and boil it down thick as tar & anoint the teter worm with this every day for several days, then make an oitment of sweet oil, the same to be made thus ; take a quart of unslacked lime, the same of muscle shells well burnt and beat, mix these together with water, so as to get half a pint of the lime water, then mix half a pint of lime water with the same quantity of sweet oil, stir it well together, until it thickens like butter, and anoint with this once or twice a day, this both eats and heals the affected part, or get some poke roots and slice them well, and then get three or four quarts of sweet cream, put them in a copper kettle, boil them a good while, anoint the tetter worm often with this, or use corrosive sublimate in water, ten grains to one pint, use this for an ointment on the tetter worm once a day, and take a purge every ten days. Or you may obtain an effectual remedy at the apothecarys shop that will cure this distressing disease, that is, get the oil of cedar wood or apple and anoint the part affected once or twice a day and you will most certainly receive a permanent cure in a few weeks.

FOR BURNS &c.,

If fever be excited by a burn, the patient should be bled and purged, with gentle laxative medicines; but the greatest dependance should be placed upon applications to be made to the part affected; as lead water, rum and water, holding the part near the fire that is affected, or immerse the part in cold water immediately and then apply wet cloths frequently wetting the same, and at the same time drink warm tea made of ginger, cloves, or pepper—continue this preparation till the inflammation subsides, then apply cold, and salted dough made of Indian corn, this is good, especially where the skin is broken—a poultice made thus: take some flaxseed, put it in a quart of water, boil it down till it begins to thicken, then add some new milk, and let it boil a little, then thicken it with a little flour, spread it on a cloth, put some fresh butter on the same, to keep it from sticking, this will draw out the fire—and at the same time heal the burn. Or get a handful of heart leaves, the same of the inside bark of elder, also sheep suet and a little fresh butter, and make an ointment, and put this on muslin and apply it to the burn. Or take unslacked lime, and slack it in common oil, or sweet oil, and take it out again as dry as you can, and make it into an ointment with oil of roses; this oil often cures, without a scar, in a little time.

THE DYSENTERY, OR BLOODY FLUX.

This disease is defined by Dr. Cullin, a contagious fever, attended with frequent slimy or bloody stools; while at the same time, the usual contents of the intestines, are for the most part retained; and with a violent griping, painful, frequent urging to go to stool. If there be a frequent desire of going to stool, especially after eating or drinking, it is considered a certain mark of this disease. It occurs in the same season that intermittent fevers do; and like them follows long dry, long moist and hot weather; sometimes it comes on with cold shivering, and other marks of fever, and in some instances, the fever attending is very violent and inflammatory: sometimes, though not so frequently, a diarrhœa is the first symptom. There is commonly a loss of appetite, frequently sickness, nausea and vomit-

ing; which are considerably proportioned to the violence of the disease. In every case where there is violent fever, the danger is considerable; when the patient
stools, he seldom breaks wind. Now to prevent this
disease from spreading, the patient should be kept very
clean, his room should be well aired, and properly
cleansed, and vinegar should be frequently poured upon a hot brick, stone, or piece of hot iron. In places
where this complaint prevails, the daily use of cold
baths; the dress of children should be carefully changed
to the state of the weather; salt meat, should be daily, but moderately used through the sickly season, and
drink tar water, morning and evening; and, when you
go among the sick, take a little of the tincture of assafœdita, ginger, or a few drops of the spirits of turpentine on sugar, or get a handful of cucumber bark, a
handful of dogwood bark, a handful of yellow poplar
bark, put them in spirits, and drink as a bitter. For the
cure of this disease, regard must be had to the degree
of fever present; for if there be great thirst, acute
pains, and a tight, though small pulse, the patient should
be bled, and if pains and other violent symptoms, continue the blood letting, repeat it every twelve or twenty-four hours, until they do yield. Pukes are sometimes proper, but they should be used only when there
is great sickness at the stomach; and if the marks of
fever, as above, be present, a puke should not be administered, until after one or more bleeding. Purges
should be frequently repeated, but they must be of the
most gentle sort, as cream of tartar, purging salts,
manna, &c. Physic grass, which is called highland
flags—take a handful and beat it, let it stand in a tum-
bler of cold water over night, drink it in the morning,
and work it off with warm water, or water gruel, but
let it be remembered, that jalap and rhubarb are not
proper in this complaint; glyster of flax seed tea, or
mutton broth, with a little tincture of opium, should be
injected, two, three, or four times, for every twenty-

four hours. If there be great heat and pain in the bowels, cold water might be injected in the form of a glyster; indeed it could do no injury, if there were no inflammatory symptoms. Opium, a dose of the tincture or a pill of the solid opium, should be given every night; and after sufficient evacuations, it might be used every six or eight hours, if necessary: cooling drinks, such as whey, flax seed tea, camomile tea, and barley water, are all proper for this purpose; and if there be much fever, cold water is a very proper drink—a decoction of gum arabic or shavings of harts-horn with spice, mutton suet boiled in milk—a decoction of blackberry brier roots, or a gruel made of a little flour prepared according to Dr. Buckhan, that is to say: take a few handfuls of fine flour, tie it up in a linen cloth, and boil it in a pot for six hours, until it becomes as hard as starch; afterwards grate it, and make it into gruel.— Either of these will be very useful; when the patient is much spent, blisters may be applied to the wrists and ancles, but not commonly, until after the fifth day. In the close of the disease, port wine, madeira or sherry wines, are proper when the fever intermits, and especially where it assumes the shape of the third day fever and ague; the bark is a very proper remedy to be given, chiefly in the fore part of the day; so is a spoonful of the juice of elder berries, two or three times a day; or take a new laid egg, and pour out the white and fill up the egg with salt, and roast it hard; then beat it to a powder, and take as much as will lay on the point of a case knife, every half hour; and let your drink be a tea of the root of black-gum, or sycamore bark tea, or take the spirits of turpentine and put on burning coals, and receive the smoke. This will stop it; and if it stops too fast, work it off with salts or castor-oil; or take dried leaves of angelico and make a tea, and drink of it, or make a tea of sweet fennel leaves, or take as much grated rhubarb as will lie on the point of a case-knife, with half as much grated nutmeg; put these in a glass of white wine, take this liying down; or take fourteen drops of laudanum, and apply to the belly a poultice of wormwood and red roses, boiled in milk, and feed on rice syrup and beef; give a spoonful of sheep suet, melted on a slow fire, a spoonful of green plantain mixed together, and take several times, and sitting in a tub of warm water, three inches deep; or take the maw of a rabbit dried to a powder, made up in doses, and taken in plantain juice; for a child, take the seeds of plantain, beat them to a powder, give a tea spoonful in red wine; or take the jaw bone of a pike, beat to a powder, take half a drachm of the powder in red wine, morning and evening; this has cured when nothing else would: or take the back bone of a beef or hog, burn until they become white, then beat them fine, boil them in new milk, and give them to drink.

THE CHOLERA MORBUS, OR PURGING AND VOMITING.

This disorder makes its appearance in warm climates as early in the season as April and May; but in colder climates, not until the middle of June, or first of July; the danger attending it, is in proportion to the heat of the weather. Children are subject to it fiom one to two weeks, until two years old. It sometimes begins with a diarrhœa, which will continue for several days without any other disorder; but most commonly violent vomiting and purging, and high fevers attend; the matter discharged from the stomach and bowels is yellow or green, the stools are sometimes slimy and mixed with blood, without any appearance of bile; sometimes the stools are as thin as water; worms are frequently voided. Whether the evacuation be billious or not, the patient seems to suffer much pain, draws up the feet, is never in one posture; the pulse weak and quick, the head very warm, the hands and feet cold; the fever

remits and returns with greater violence every evening.
The head is some times so much affected, that the patient not only becomes delirious, but will rave and try
to scratch or bite the parent or nurse. The belly, and
sometimes the face and limbs swell—has great thirst in
every stage—the eyes appear languid and hollow,
sleeps with them half closed, so gieat is the insensibili-
ty of his eyes, that flies light upon them while
open, and do not excite the least motion in the eye-lids.
Sometimes the vomiting continues without the purging,
but more commonly the purging remains without the
vomiting. Through the whole course of the disorder,
the stools are, sometimes large, emitting a very disagreeable smell; at other times there are scanty stools,
without smell, like the food or drink taken in by the
child. This disorder is sometimes fatal in a few days;
and in some cases, even in twenty-four hours—much
depends on the state of the weather, one cool day generally abates; the time or violence of its duration,
varies frequently from a few days to six weeks, or two
months; when it is of long standing, and tending to
death, there is commonly great wasting of the patient's
flesh; the bones will sometimes come through the skin.
Towards the close of the disease, there appears purple
spots on the skin, with hiccough, convulsions, ghastly
countenance and sore mouth; when those last appearances come on the case generally becomes incurable.
The following remarks may help to guard against mis-
takes in this disorder: It is sometimes thought to be
the effect of teething; but as it comes on in a particular season of the year, this mistake may be avoided.
It is true, however, that it is rendered more violent
when it happens to seize on children in the time of
teething. It is sometimes attributed to worms; but
although worms are frequently voided in this fever,
they are never the cause of it. It has been considered
the effect of eating summer fruits; but where children
can get ripe fruit at pleasure, it seldom occurs; and in-

deed ripe fruits taken moderately, have a considerable tendency to prevent it. On the whole, it may be considered a species of the billious fever, and may be cured as follows: Give a puke to evacuate the bile from the stomach; this may be done by a dose of ipecacuana or tartar emetic, and it should be repeated as often as there is vomiting of bile. In every stage of the disorder, the bowels should then be purged with manna, castoroil or magnesia; but rubarb is not a proper remedy until the fever is subdued in some considerable degree. If, however, the puking and purging have continued until there is good reason to believe that the offending matter has been thrown off by the natural efforts, the pukes and purges must be omitted, and instead of them a few drops of the tincture of opium may be given in a chalk julip, say prepared chalk or crabs claws, eight grains to twenty, tincture of opium, half a dose, or three to four, cinnamon water or peppermint tea at discretion; syrup, as much as may be suficient to make it pleasant, to be given every three or four, or six hours; sometimes a few drops of spirits of harts-horn will be a useful addition to the above julep. Small blisters might be applied to the region of the stomach, or to the wrists and ancles. Mint and mallow teas, or a tea of blackberry brier roots, infused in cold water; a decoction of shavings of hartshorn, or a solution of gum arabic, or a tea of the pith of Sassafras-wood, steeped in warm water, with the addition of a little mint or cinnamon, either of these articles may be prepared and used as drink. To compose the stomach or bowels, glysters made of flax seed tea or mutton soup, or starch dissolved in water. Either of those, with the addition of a few drops of the tincture of opium, may be frequently injected. Plasters of venice treacles, where it can be had, or flannels wet with a strong infusion of bitter herbs, in warm spirits or madeira wine, might be applied to the stomach; or what might be still more convenient, a cloth folded so

as to be two or three inches square, might be wet with
the tincture of opium, and applied as before. As soon
as the violent symptoms are subdued, give bark in the
form of decoction, or in substance, to which may be
added a little nutmeg; or if bark be offensive to the
patient, use port wine, or claret in its stead. At this
stage, it will be proper to indulge the child in any particular article of strong food. The patient may happen to crave salted or dried fish, salt meat, butter or
rich gravies, and even the strongest cheese. Another
remedy when there is great pain, is the warm bath; and
it would be still more effectual, if wine were used instead of water. It is also probable, that a cold bath,
a few times repeated, would be an excellent remedy in
the recovering stage of the disease; it will be found
very beneficial, to carry the child out to breathe a fresh
country air. In places where this complaint prevails,
the following particulars will probably prevent the
daily use of the cold bath: The dress of children should
be carefully accommodated to the state and changes of
the weather; salted meat should be daily, but moderately used through the sickly season; good sound wine
may be given them in portions adapted to their age;
from a tea spoonful to a half a wine glass full, at the
discretion of the parents: particular regard should be
had to cleanliness, both with respect to their skin and
clothing. Lastly, persons living in sickly towns, ought
to be especially attentive to all these dangerous complaints; and where it can be done, they should remove
their children to the country, before the sickly season.
I have cured many with bowman root, which is called
by some, Indian physic. Boil a good handful in two
quarts of water, to a pint, let them drink freely of that,
and drink warm water to work it off; or take a table
spoonful of beet puccoon root, a spoonful of fennel
seed, a spoonful of mountain birch bark, beat it fine;
you may let this stand for time of need; this decoction
is to be put in a quart of cider; a child of two or three

years of age, is to take a tea spoonful once or twice a day, and so on according to the age; to a grown person, a table spoonful, not to eat hog meat nor milk.

THE PLEURISY—THE SYMPTOMS.

This comes on like other fevers. It generally begins with chillness and shivering, which are followed by heat, thirst and restlessness; to these succeeds a violent pricking pain, in one of the sides among the ribs, sometimes the pain extends towards the back bone; sometimes towards the fore part of the breast, and at other times towards the blades; the pain is generally most violent when the patient draws in his breath—if he holds his breath as long as he can, he cannot fetch his breath without coughing. The pulse in this disease is commonly quick and hard; the urine is high colored, and if blood is let, it is covered with a tough crust, or buffy coat; the patient's spittle is at first thin, but afterwards it becomes grosser, and is often streaked with blood; there is generally a violent pain in the side, and high fevers, changing from place to place, and sometimes in the head, with a shortness of breath, that you will appear to be choking, and generally weakens the patient fast, and often turns to the third day fever and ague. Make a decoction of nettles and apply the boiled herbs as hot as you can bare it to the pain; or beat brimstone fine, or the flour of sulphur, mix up the white of two eggs, and put to the pain; let your diet be light, and cooling; let your drink be whey, water gruel, barley water, hysop tea, sharpened with vinegar, or lemon juice and water. If the spitting stops suddenly, take a little vomit. like camphorated vinegar, syrup, elder berries, raspberries or straw berries, this is good to cleanse the lungs; bleeding is oftentimes wonderful good, sometimes roasted apples or currents is good.

. There is a bastard pleurisy·and a true one, that is to·
say, an inflammation in the ribs, attended with little, or.
no fever; the.Pleurisy is attended with a violent fever·
and pains in the sides, the pulse remarkably hard; he
may take a strong decoction of sennaca snake root,
which is called by some rattle snake root, or a spoonful
of pleursy root, also called butterfly root, and then
cover up warm in bed; any kind of warm dilutary
drinks, or take a handful of dried poke berries, a handful of saw dust of light wood, a handful of diied horehound, a spoonful of brimstone, a half spoonful of saltpeter, a spoonful of beat rattle snake root, to a quart of·
whiskey, (rye whiskey is the best) take a table.spoon-
full twice a day; beware of taking cold, or going out in
the dew, or after sunset; blisters are good when the pain·
continues. If.the body be bound take some of the bark
of white walnut and elder roots, boil them, take out the
roots and put in some saltpeter, boil this to a thick mass,
and form it into pills, and take them when needed.—
These pills will neither leave you bound nor gripe you,
if the sweat does not·break, it is good to put a little
dogwood bark in, this decoction of pills, that is, the
white walnut pills.

THE SCARLET FEVER.

This fever, like the foregoing, depends on a specific
contagation; it comes on with chilliness and sickness
at the stomach, and vomiting. These symptoms are
specially characteristic of the disease: there are in
some cases a swelling of the throat, and difficulty of
speaking, swallowing and breathing—sometimes there
is a squeaking voice, and ulcers in the throat, which are
in some instances deep and covered with white brown
or black sloughs; a thick mucus is discharged from the
nose, sometimes from the beginning, but more com-

monly coming on about the fifth day ; an eruption appears on the skin, sometimes preceding, sometimes
following the ulcers and swelling of the throat ; in some
the eruption is confined to the outside of the throat and
breast ; in others wholly to the limbs : in some it appears on the second and third day, and never afterwards ; in some it appears with the sore throat, and
perhaps in others without it—the bowels are generally
regular but some have a diarrhœa. This fever is moderately inflammatory, and differs from the malignant
fever or putrid sore throat. The eruption in this fever is of a deeper red color, and is more smooth, the
skin being more hot and dry ; the skin peels off in the
close of the fever. It is not so dangerous as the putrid
sore throat, it commonly goes off with the swelling
of the hands and feet ; and lastly, it frequently appears
in summer and dry weather. Again, this fever may
be distinguished from a common inflammation of the almonds, &c., called quinsey, by the following remarks :
the appearance of ulcers, in common quinsey is confined to the almonds, &c.—a strong, full and tense
pulse attend an inflammatory quinsey, always admitting the use of the lancet. A common quinsey is not
attended with external redness. The remedies for the
scarlet fever, puking, ipecacuana and colomel combined
as the putrid sore throat ; wash the mouth with
barley water, or very thin gruel, to which should be
added a little vinegar and honey, if convenient, a portion of the tincture of myrrh ; sixty or eighty drops of
the tincture of myrrh might be added to half an ounce
of the gruel, &c., or if the myrrh cannot be had, as
much calomel might be added instead of it, as may be
sufficient to turn it of a whitish color. I have found
great benefit from frequently washing the mouth and
throat well with the following mixture : take salt peter,
half an ounce, Borax, one quarter of an ounce, the
whole to be dissolved in one pint of water, and sweetened with honey. I have used it successfully in a num-

ber of cases without any other topical operation—snuff
may be used about the fifth day to excite a running at
the nose. Towards the close of the disease, wine and
water, or wine and whey, may be used to such extent
only as to keep up a gentle perspiration. When ever
the swelling of the extremeties takes place, a dose of
calomel may be repeated. It is worthy of observation,
that this disease can be communicated before it can be
known to be present in any case ; it is therefore unnecessary to remove children out of the family where
it makes its appearance. Some are of opinion that
scarlet fever might be prevented by using occasional
does of rheubarb ; this remedy is worthy of trial. Children are mostly subject to it.

THE MESENTERIC FEVER.

There is another disease, which has its principal seat
in the intestinal glands, and may therefore be properly
admissable in this place. It is fever excited by obstructions in the mesentary ; from which circumstances it
has its name. Children are subject to it from infancy
up to the age of three or four, and even six or eight
years. This fever remits, and some times has irregular intermission, attended with a loss of appetite swelled belly and pain in the bowels, and has often been mistaken for worms. If, therefore, the usual remedies
should fail, the child will sooner or later be affected with
indigeston, costiveness, or purging, irregular appetite,
flushed cheeks, or total loss of color, impaired strength
and spirits, remitting fever, a hard belly, and emacia-
ted limbs. These symptoms, will therefore, sufficiently
specify the disease ; it frequently follows measels, and
other eruptive fevers. Children that are confined to
coarse and unwholesome food ; are badly clothed ; not
kept sufficiently clean, specify the disease. It frequent-

ly follows measels, also those who are neglected so as not to receive sufficient exercise, are most subject to its attack. Hence, the negro children of the southern states frequently perish with this fever. When any symptoms of this distructive disease presents themselves, enquiry should made into the manner of feeding, clothing and cleaning the child; and every error in the articles must be corrected; and if the patient has not too long labored under its influence, frequent purging with calomel will of itself perform a cure. In more advanced stages of this complaint, it would be best to call in the aid of a physician; but where this is impractible, proceed to give the following bolus three times a week. Take calomel, two grains; ipecacuana, from a half to one grain; nutmeg or ginger powdered (six grains) to be mixed up in honey syrup, for one dose for a child from two to four years old; fifteen or twenty drops of antimonial wine may be given the intervening nights where the calomel is not used. Having continued those remedies till the fever is removed, hardness of the belly subsided, &c., then the strength of the patient should be restored, by the use of the bark, steel, cold bath, bitters, &c., Gentle exercise, friction, light nourishing food &c. All greasy or fat articles should be avoided as also those preparations of pastry, which are often of a clammy nature.

THE WHOOPING COUGH OR CHIN COUGH.

This disease commonly falls upon a whole neighborhood about the same, and is therefore, said to be epedemic. It is manifestly contagious; it affects persons but once in their lives. Children therefore, are most commonly the subjects of it; sometimes, however, it occurs in persons considerably advanced in life, but grown persons, and those who are elderly in proportion

to their age, are less, liable to be affected than children,
and youths growing up.   This complaint at first, puts
on the appearance of a common cold ; and Dr. Cullin,
makes mention of instances which never assumed any
other shape, than that of a cold, although they · were
obviously the effects of this contagion.   But this is not
commonly the case ; geneially in the second week or
at most the third, the convulsive motions which gives
the name to this disease, manifestly shows itself, and is
commonly called the hoop ; this hoop, together with the
circumstances of the general spread of the disorder,
sufficiently distinguishes the chin cough. Dr. Darwin
says it consists in an inflamation of the membrane, which
lines the vessels of the lungs ; the whole of them are
probably not infected at the same : but the contagious
inflammation continues gradually to creep on the membrane—this opinion seems to account very well for its
long continuance—which is from one month, to three
and sometimes much longer.   This complaint, is not
usually classed among febrile disorders, but a fever
may generally be perceived to attend it during some
part of the day, especially in weak patients, and a general iflammation of the lungs frequently supervenes
and destroys great numbers of children. Except the
lancet, or four or six leeches, be immediately and repeatedly used, when the child has permanent difficulty
of breathing, (which continues between the coughing
fits,) unless the blood be taken, he dies in a few days ; if
the inflammation of the lungs during this permanent difficulty of breathing, the hooping cough abates or quite
ceases.   Many have been deceived by this c rcumstance,
unfortunately supposing the child to be better.   But after once or twice bleeding, the cough returns, which is
then a good symptom, as the child possessing the power
to cough, is relieved, and once more breaths with ease.
The remedies in this disease are gentle vomits of tartar emetic ; this article should be given in small doses,
frequently repeated, till it produces the intended effect ;

mild purges repeated, till they produce a looseness in the bowels; and open blisters to be frequently repeated; they may be applied to one or both sides of the breast. Warm bath: this is an excellent remedy where the cough is violent, and the child much exhausted. In every instance where there is difficulty of breathing between the fits of coughing, the only safe remedy, is copious bleeding; if this be neglected or omitted, the child may die; young children should lie with their heads and shoulders raised, and should be constantly watched day and night, to prevent them from strangling in the cough. A little bow of whale bone, or elastic wood, should be used to extract the phlegm out of the mouths of infants. The application of a handkerchief to their mouths when in the act of coughing, might suffocate them. After the disease has continued some weeks, and especially if the patient be much reduced, the following dose, calculated for a child, three or four years old, may be useful: say calomel, one sixth part of a grain, rhubarb two grains, to be combined and repeated twice a day; but opium will be very pernicious as long as blood letting is proper.— Towards the close of the complaint, all feeble patients should be daily carried out on horse back. This is a most excellent remedy.

THE MEASLES.

This disease is epidemic; it depends on a specific contagion, and occurs most frequently in children; no age, however, is exempted from it, if the person has not been subjected to it before. It commonly first appears in the month of January, and ceases after the middle of the summer; but by various accidents, it may be produced at other times of the year. The symptoms are as follows: the disease always begins

with a cold chill, which is soon followed by the usual
symptoms of fever, thirst, heat, loss of appetite, anxiety,
sickness and vomiting, and these are more or less considerable in different cases : in many instances, the fever for the first two days is inconsiderable ; and in different cases, sometimes it is violent from the beginning,
and always becomes violent before the eruption appears. This fever is always attended with hoarseness ;
with a frequent hoarse, dry cough, and often with
some difficulty of breathing ; the eyes inflamed and
watery ; there is a discharge from the nose, with frequent sneezing ; in most instances the patient is drow-
sy in the beginning ; the eruption commonly appears
on the fourth day : first on the face, and successively
on the lower parts of the body. It shows itself first in
small red points, which collect together in clusters
on the face, and where, by the sense of touch, they
are easily perceived to be a little elevated ; but they
can scarcely be felt on other parts of the body.—
The redness of the face continues, and sometimes increases for two days. On the third day, the vivid redness is changed to a brownish red, and in a day or two
more, the eruption entirely disappears, and is followed
by a branny scale. During the whole time of the
eruption, the face appears full, but not much swelled,
sometimes the fever disappears as soon as the eruption
takes place. But this is seldom the case, more commonly it continues, or is increased after the eruption ;
and in some instances, even after the branny scales appear. As long as the fever exists in a considerable degree, the cough continues, and that generally with an
increase of the difficulty of breathing. Sometimes an
inflammation of the lungs takes place : this is a very serious circumstance when it occurs, and ought to be
specially observed. All the above symptoms admit of
very great variation ; and in some caseses, there will
be in addition to the soreness of the throat ; spitting
blood mixed with phlegm coughed up ; gripes, diarrhœa

and bloody stools. I suppose that fourteen days inter-
vene between the time of receiving the infection, and
the appearance of the disease. It may be well to observe, that the eruption does not invariably appear on
the third or fourth day, but varies even to the eighth;
neither does the eruption disappear invariably on a
certain day, nor in an unchanging manner; nor is it
always followed by the branny scales. The lever attending the measles, is in most instances, of the inflammatory kind ; but by improper management or neglect
as well as by the predisposing circumstances attending
the patient, it may assume a different form. The remedies to be employed in this disorder : blood letting :
this is always necessary when there is a full pulse, attended with great pain and violent cough ; and that
too in every stage of the disease, whether before or after the eruption takes place ; or even after the eruption
has entirely disappeared. Vomits ; a dose of ippecac-
uanha will generally remove the sickness at the stomach, soothing drinks such as barley water,balm or flax seed
tea, cider or vinegar mixed with water, or apple water,
dried cherry water, &c. This moistens the throat, and
affords much relief. Blisters after sufficient evacuations
by bleeding ; otherwise blisters may be applied to the
neck and sides ; they prevent injury to the lungs.—
Opiates ; if the pulse be not soft and the patient labors
under the distressing symptoms of the diarrhœa and
cough, opium may be used, not only at night, but at
any time during the day. In most instances, if the patient be kept cool, and take opening and cooling
drinks &c ; if he be bled when the symptoms are violent, as also about the time the measles disappear, or-
when the branny scale presents itself, and if his bowels be opened on the third and fourth day of the eruption with cream of tartar, flour of sulphur manna or
the like ; little else will be wanting, especially in children's cases. Here, let it be particularly observed,
that in every instance, where the eruption seems to

take place with difficulty, and where the pulse is $\frac{2}{2}$ full, and with other marks of great fever; all spirituous liquors and other heating medicines, are highly perni- cious; in such cases frequent bleeding would be much more proper. It may be useful also, to observe, that there is a fever which sometimes takes place du- ring the prevalence of the measles, very much resem- bling that disease, assuming the appearance of an erup- tion. But persons are still liable to take the true measles, after having been subjected to this disease : it is some- times attended with symptoms of the croup, that is to say, the hives ; and in that case, treatment must be the same, as if croup were the original disorder, in all other respects the remedies useful in measles might be employed in this kind of fever. Patients when re- covering from the measles, are frequently subject to diarrhœa; this uncomfortable symptom, may be re- moved by moderate doses of opium, frequently repeat- ed. The drinks recommended above will be of great use. Sore eyes sometimes follow the measles ; these are to be cured by blistering the temples, and back of the neck, and washing the eyes with weak solution of white vitriol. A cough and fever frequently attend for sometime after the eruption disappears: these are to be relieved by a vegetable diet : warmth, and gently riding out in the fresh air. When the measles are ex- pected, it will be found benfiecial to prepare for them, by living chiefly on milk and vegetable diet, and by avoiding every kind of spirits.

A CANCER.

A cancer is often thought light of, but it is a grow- ing evil; it is like putting a little fire into dry stubble : you may stop it when you are a head of it, but when that gets a head of you, it is a bad chance. When a cancer first comes it is like the body of a spider; then as it increases, the roots run off like a spider's legs; then if you can conquer the body before the legs can support themselves, the cancer is done, by eating or cutting them out. Some think to eat a cancer away when it gets to a stand, and by that means put their fire medicines, which causes the cancer to eat as fast as the medicine, and inflame in a short time considerably. When a cancer comes first, it scarcely has any colour; often times it is like a lump in the skin; after sometime there rises a kind of blister, and sometimes with yel-low water and at other times clear water; then there is little shooting pains at times from it, but no great misery, at times there will be a kind of itching, and at other times the itching will in a great measure go away. So it works for a long time, and sometimes it eats very fast. I have given some of the most prominent symptoms of this painful disease. I shall now proceed to give some of the best remedies that have ever yet been known, for the removal of the same. In the first place, get a handful of the inside bark of white oak, and make a strong ooze, and wash the cancer well before you apply the salve, every time; then put your salve on a patch, and put it on the cancer twice a day, the salve is made thus:— Get a handful of the inside bark of red oak, and a double handful of persimmon bark, the same of the bark of the roots of dogwood, the same of the bark of sassafras roots, and also one hand ful of the roots of dew berry; put these articles all together; and boil them slowly about twelve hours, then take out the barks and roots, strain it, then put it back again and boil it down as thick as tar. This is the finest salve that I ever knew, when the cancer has come to a stand, or matters, for there has been many cured with this preparation, that were proclaimed incurable. It takes out the inflammation and turns the cancer to a matter, &c. It would be good to put now and then a poultice made of the following articles to wit:—Get a

double handful of sassafras bark of the root, the same
of the root of dogwood, the same of sumac roots, boil
these well about half a day, take out the barks, and
manage it the same way as the other medicines above.
You may burn alum and take an equal quantity of copperas and blue stone well beat together, and sprinkle
in the cancer, and then put on the salve. But if the
cancer be not broke, make a sheet of lead, beat very
thin, and pricked full of fine holes and applied to the
place; purges should be taken every third or fourth
day, and rub the cancer every now and then with spirits of hartshorn mixed with oil; or apply red onions
bruised; or make a plaster of rock alum, vinegar and
honey, equal quantities, with wheat flour; change it
every twelve hours; this often cures—you may drink
plentifully of tar water. Here is a kind of pot-ash that
I have found to be of great advantage, that is to slice up
a good chance of poke roots and put them in a pot
over a hot fire till they become ashes, then clean your
hearth and put an equal quantity of black ash bark
white hickory bark and also yellow sarsaparilla, burn
these to ashes, and let them soak to a strong lye, then
boil the lye down to a powder; this powder is wonderful to eat cancers, cankers, and old running sores.
There is an herb commonly called beach drop, when
dried and beaten to a powder, and mixed with tar, is
a fine salve to eat away cancers. Or take half a pint of
small beer, when it boils, dissolve in it an ounce and a
half of bees wax, then put in an ounce of hog's lard,
and boil them together; when it is cold, pour the beer
from it, and apply it by spreading it upon white leather, renew it every other day, it brings out great blotches; wash it with an ooze made of dogwood bark, black
oak bark and sassafras bark: or get an equal quantity
of blue vitriol and white vitriol, as much red precipitate, as of either of the quantities of vitriol, beat well
together and sprinkle in the sore, and boil slippery elm,
and thicken it well with sweet milk and flour, and put

on as a poultice or salve, and wash it now and then
with the elixir vitriol, and to heal it, dissolve the sugar
of lead in spring water and thicken it with flour and
honey, and use this as a salve; or beat twenty grains
of copperas, five of calomel, well mixed together, and
sprinkle it in the sore.

DYSPEPSIA, OR INDIGESTION.

This is a complaint very prevalent in our country:
it is not only confined to the aged; but to the middle
aged, both women and men are subject to this disorder,
The causes are very numerous which produce this complaint, it frequently comes from colds, hard study, and
a sedentary life, exposure, hard lifts, &c., the symptoms
generally connected with this disease are the following:
The stomach becomes deranged, the regular functions
are much impaired, a tingling in the flesh, a weakness
in the eyes, swiming in the head, beating in the pit of
the stomach, frequently belching up sour wind, rumbling
noise in the bowels, pain in the side, sometimes in the
arms, then in the shoulder and in the shoulder blade, roar-
ing in the ears, restlessness, burning in the stomach, frequently the patient belches up what he eats, generally a bad taste in the mouth, particularly in the morning
sometimes the appetite is very good, then rather limited, the bowels generally costive, though at times rather loose, with a general depression of spirits.

In the treatment of this unpleasant disease, the first
thing necessary is to purge the blood, and give regular
tone to the stomach and bowels, owing to the irreglar-
ity of the blood, and the debility of the same, there is
a quantity of slime and mucus collects in the stomach,
which is necessary to be worked off by mild purges,
rather of a stimulons nature. In order to purge the
blood, and give tone to the system, get a peck of horse

radish root, the same of sassafras, the same of the root
of wild cherry, the same of burdock, put them in a pot
add ten gallons of water, boil it down to two gallons,
take it out and strain it, then put it back again in the
pot, then add a half table spoonful of salt petre or refined nitre, add two pounds of sugar, one quart of
French Brandy, boil it down to one gallon, it is then fit
for use; the patient should take from a half to a table
spoonful three times a day, abstain from the use of
strong diet while using the above medicines. Take five
ounces of magnesia, the same of charcoal, the same of
mandrake or may apple root, pulverise them all fine together; the patient should take half a table spoonful
every third night with the white of an egg. This medicine will have a tendency of regulating the bowels,
and it will produce that regularity on the liver that is
necessary in dyspeptic cases, and it will also work off
the mucus and slime that is collected there. In order
to strengthen the stomace, the patient should take a
small portion of the oil of Juniper, also the tincture of
quinine; the patient should frequently drink pennyroyal
tea, a little weak lye at times is also necessary, when there
is any swelling in the stomach or much burning, take a
small pill of beefs gall every night until it subsides, if
there is much wind on the stomach, take ten drops of
the oil of peppermint, two or three times a day, while
using any of these medicines the patient should live on
the most limited kind of diet, use nothing that is the
least strong, and at the same time avoid taking cold or
getting wet, if the weather is pleasant the patient should
travel through the country, and avoid reading or any
thing that is calculated to agitate the mind.

It is too frequently the case, that persons who are
afflicted with this melancholy disease, or are apt to be
in the habit of studying a great deal, and frequently
think there is no cure for them. I well recollect a case
of a gentleman who came to me for medicine, after taking it about two or three weeks, he returned again

and said my medicine was too weak for his case, I told him to try some other Physician awhile, accordingly he did so, the doctor salivated him severely. So soon as he got able to ride he returned again. He said that the doctor had eat up his liver with calomel, that he had spit up great mouthfulls of his liver frequently, that he believed that it was all gone, and there was none left, that there was a great vacancy in his breast that he never felt before. Being in my shop, shutting one door and at the same time telling him to sit down, and beginning to open his waistcoat before, and having a knife in my hand — said he doctor what are you going to do, I informed him that I intended to open a place on his side, to see if his liver was all gone; stop said he doctor one minute if you please, until I see if my horse is at the rack; no sooner had he got to his horse and on him, than he started and it would have taken a score of men of sound livers to have caught him.

PHTHISIC, OR PULMONARY CONSUMPTION.

This disease is generally accompanied with a debility of the whole system—pain in the side or chest, particularly after walking or speaking, with a tickling cough which proves most troublesome in the morning; in an advanced stage, purulent expectoration ensues, with hectic fever and diarrhœa; pulmonary consumption does not often occur until after the age of puberty, but in some cases it is evidently formed before that period. Women are more subject to it than men, as well from their going more slightly clothed, as from the greater delicacy of their organization. The causes which predispose to this disease are very numerous—the following, however, are most general: hereditary disposition, particular formation of the body, obvious by a long neck, permanent shoulders, and narrow chest, scrofulous diathesis, indicated by a fine clear skin, fair hair, delicate rosy complexion, large thick upper lip, weak voice and great sensibility. This disorder comes by many causes ; wet feet, night air, wet clothes, over-heats, sudden changes of weather, and particularly women not taking care when their terms are on them, which causes them to abate, corrupts their blood and settles on their lungs, and turns to a deep consumption, if not brought on by regular means, it is bad for shoe-makers, seamsters, and such as lean on the breast : this disease generally begins with a dry tickling cough, which continues frequently a long time before it takes life, at other times it is of a short duration. Those that have this complaint some days, have a craving appetite, and then at other times, have scarcely any. They cough mostly in the morning, and oftentimes soreness and oppression in the breast, a shortness of breath, weakness in the knees, the spittle is at first of a sweetish fainty taste. Then as the disease progresses, the spittle is of a whitish frothy color, the patient is often sad, the thirst is often great, the pulse quick and small, at other times full and hard, at this time there is generally a dull heavy feeling, stretching or gaping at times, which if not checked enters into the second stage, the spittle that was before of a whitish frothy color, is become a greenish color, and at times streaked with blood, often a swimming in the head, mostly after a spell of coughing or eating. There is a kind of hectic fever takes place in this stage; and night sweats now it enters into the third stage. There is a burning heat in the palms of the hands, a looseness in the bow-els, at this time the end of the nails turn upwards, the swelling of the feet and legs, and sinking of the eyes, difficulty of swallowing and coldness of the feet ; when these last symptoms come on, the patient may find a physician for the soul, but none for the body ; the rem-edy or treatment—take one peck of horehound, the same of elecampane, the same of comfrey, the same of the bark of the root of yellow poplar, the same of ground-ivy, the same of penneroyal, put the ingredients all together, boil them all in fifteen gallons of water, down to three gallons, take out the liquid and strain it—to this add half a gallon of honey or molasses, add one tea spoonful of the oil of annis, one quart of old rye whiskey, boil it again down to one gallon, then cork it up in a jug or bottle, let it stand for three days, it is then fit for use, the patient may take from a tea spoonful, to half a table spoonful three times a day, mixed in a few drops of sweet oil, or new fresh butter, while using this medicine, eat no hog meat nor sweet milk—this medicine will purify the blood, and produce an expectoration from the lungs. If the bowels are costive, pulverize the inside bark of wild cherrytree, of this the patient may take a half a table spoonful every third or fourth night, in a little honey; if the cough should be dry and hard, drink freely of a tea made of the inside bark of prickly-ash, when the cough abates put one quart of rum to a half a pound of rosin, stir it well until the rosin is disolved, add three ounces of loaf sugar, one ounce of peruvian bark, let it stand for two or three days, the patient should then take a tea spoonful three or four times a day, in a little water. If the patient should continue to be weak, take one quart of vinegar, two tea spoonfuls of elixir-vitriol, one ounce of rhubarb, one ounce of orange pealings, half an ounce of pulverized columbo root, shake this well together for two or three days, take a tea spoonful three or four times a day. If there should be night sweats, take a tea spoonful of sweet spirits of nitre every two or three hours until it abates, if the patient should have a diarrhœa or dysentery, take two ounces of angelico seed, the same of coriander seed, half an ounce of gum kino, put this in one quart of spirits, boil it down slow to one pint, strain it, take from one tea spoonful to a small table spoonful three times a day.

´HYDROTHORAX, OR DROPSY OF THE CHEST.

Oppression of breathing, particularly on motion, and when in a horizontal posture, difficulty of lying on the side where effusion does not exist, sudden startings from sleep, with anxiety, palpitations at the heart, irregularity of the pulse, cough, occasional syncype, paleness of visage, anasarcous swelling of the lower extremities, thirst, and diminution of urine, which is high colored, and on cooling desposits a pink or red sediment, are the characteristic symptoms of hydrothorax; but the one which is more decisive than all the rest, is a sensation of water being perceived in the chest, by the patient, on certain motions of the belly, or as if the heart were moving in a fluid. By percussion with the hand upon the chest, when the patient is in an erect position, and also by pressure upon the abdomen, which considerably aggravates the sense of suffocation for the moment, as well as the other symptoms which attend on hydrothorax, we may be able in many cases, clearly to ascertain the accumulation of water in the chest. The former is strongly reccommended as a test by Covissart, and the latter by Bichat, both of them being men of eminence. By combining both means, we may be able to determine more decisively, than by adopting either singly. The disease with which hydrothorax is most likely to be confounded, are, empyema, angina pectoris, asthma, and organic affections of the heart, or aneurismal dilations of the large vessels connected with it; but by a close attention to the symptoms which have been pointed out under these heads, we shall be able to distinguish between them with tolerable accuracy.

The causes which gave rise to the disease are pretty much the same with those which are productive of the other species of dropsy. In some cases it exists without any other kind of dropsical affection being present, but it prevails very often as a part of more universal

dropsy. Hydrothorax is frequently a disease of advanced life, and like other dropsical affections, it often
succeeds dibility, however induced. It chiefly attacks
males who have addicted themselves to free living,
especially to potations of any intoxicating liquor.—
Suce as have long suffered from gout and asthma, are
particularly liable to it. It frequently takes place to a
considerable degree, before it becomes very perceptible ; and its presence is not readily known : the symptoms, like those of hydrocephalus, not being always
very distinct. In some instances, the water is collected in both cases of the pleura, but at other times it is
only in one. Sometimes it is lodged in the pericardium
alone; but for the most part, it only appears there when
at the same time a collection is present in one or both
cavities of the thorax. Sometimes the water is effused
in the cellular texture of the lungs, without any being
deposited in the cavity of the thorax. In a few cases
the water that is collected is enveloped in small cysts
of a membranous nature, known by the name of hy-
datids, which seem to float in the cavity; but more
frequently they are connected with, and attached to a
particular part of the internal surface of the pleura.—
Hydrothorax often comes on with a sense of uneasiness
at the lower end of the sternum, accompanied by a
difficulty of breathing, which is much increased by any
exertion or motion, and which is always most considerable during night, when the body is in a horizontal
posture. Along with these symptoms there is a cough,
that is at first dry, but which after a time, is attended
with an expectoration of thin mucus. There is likewise a paleness of the complexion, and an anasarcous
swelling of the feet and legs, together with a considerable degree of thirst, and a diminished flow of urine;
occasionally the face swells, and pits upon pressure ;
especially in the morning, and these signs of disease
are accompanied by debility and loss of flesh. Under
these appearances, we have just grounds to suspect that

there is a collection of water in the chest. The symptoms which have been described, gradually increase, but their progress is slow, and a considerable time elapses before the disorder is fully formed. The difficulty of breathing at length becomes excessive. The patient can seldom remain in a recumbent posture for any time, and the head and upper part of the trunk must be supported almost erect. The sleep is frequently interrupted on a sudden by alarming dreams, out of which the patient quickly starts up in bed, with a sense of impending suffocation. Convulsive efforts of the muscles subservient to respiration, resembling an attack of spasmodic asthma, with violent palpitations of the heart generally accompany the paroxysm which are also frequently exerted by the most trifling voluntary motion, or by a fit of coughing. When afflicted with these distressing symptoms, the patient is under the neessity of continuing erect, with his mouth open, and he betrays the utmost anxiety for fresh air. His face and extremities are cold ; the pulse with little excption is feeble, irregular, intermits in a degree seldom experienced in other disorders, and a pain, or sensation of numbness frequently extends itself from the heart, towards the insertion of the deltoid muscle of one or both arms. Excepting a livid hue of the lips and cheeks, the countenance is pale, and indicates a peculiar anxiety and ghastliness of appearance, and together with the upper parts of the body is usually covered with a profuse clammy sweat. Drowsiness, coma, or delirium, occasioned by the difficult transmission of the blood through the lungs, and want of sleep frequently attends the latter periods of hydrothorax, and from the same cause the expectoration is sometimes bloody. Now and then a sensation of water floating about can be distinctly perceived by the patient, on any sudden change of posture. In the treatment of hydrothorax, it should be attended with a great deal of care and caution.

Emetics and diuretics, with respect to the emetics the tincture of ipecacuahana, from a tea spoonful to half a table spoonful should be used in a little warm water for a few times in succession, then take the following preparation, take three ounces of the cream of tartar, the same of pulverized egg shells, the egg shells should be parched, ground and made as fine as flour, take the same quantity of pulverised angelica, (the angelica is to be ground in the same way as the egg shells) the same quantity of spignard roots prepared in the same way as the above — these should all be well mixed together, and the patient should take from a tea spoonful to a half a table spoonful three times a day; this course of treatment should be pursued for six or eight days, it will have a tendency of carrying of the water by the bowels and urine. It will probably be necessary for the patient to rest three or four days, and during the intervals, strengthening and mild tonics should be used freely—then the same course should be pursued again, until the water appears to be entirely discharged from the stomach and thorax; a strong tea made of smart weed, sarsaparilla and horsemint, equally combined, should be freely used every night at bed time, just as the patient is lying down. If the bowels should become costive, the patient should take one pound of may apple root, the same of butternut (white walnut) the same of wild elder root, this should be boiled in a half gallon of water down to half a pint, of this preparation the patient should take a tea spoonful as necessity may require. Should there be any swelling of the extremities, the following solution should be used externally all over the body, every night warmed by fire. Two ounces of the sugar of lead the same of sulphuric ether, the same of the oil of pennyroyal, the same of the spirits of turpentine; this should be well mixed in one quart of alcohol, this forms one of the best external applications that I have ever used in those cases — to carry down the swelling and general inflamations of the system externally. Should the pulse be quick and hard, a little blood may be taken every two or three days. Blisters may at times be drawn on the ancles, where there is any great excitement existing. So soon as the thorax appear to be relieved from the water, the following preparation may be used, which will give tone to the bowels, and will produce that regular action, which nature requires. Get one pound of the inside bark of sycamore, the same of black berry brier root, the same of red oak, the same of yellow poplar, the same of spice wood root, the same of green plantain, the same of black haw root, the same of black gum root, the same of peach tree leaves, or rhubarb, or may apple root — these ingredients are all put together and boiled in four gallons of cider, weak vinegar, or water, down to one quart, after this is strained, there should be added one quart of molasses, the same of Peach brandy or rum, twenty grains pulverised refined nitre, ten grains of quinine, this preparation well mixed together, the patient should take from one tea spoonful to one table spoonful three times a day, this may be increased or decreased according to the nature of the case. Wine and barks may also be used at times, with any palliative that is calculated to strengthen the system. I have laid down in the first place the general symptoms of the complaint, and the treatment which should be very strictly attended to, and if this course of treatment should be strictly attended to, the patient may be relieved nine times out of ten by the efficacy of the preceeding remedies.

HEMORHAGE OR FLOODING.

Get a handful of common cherry tops, the same of black berry brier roots, the same of white oak tops, put those in two quarts of water, and boil it down to a pint, and let the patient drink of this according to the emergency of the case.

I never have known this medicine to fail. Or you may take a small quantity of green plantain bruise it, obtain the juice and give the patient a table spoonful every half hour until an abatement of this distressing complaint takes place. Or get a handful of service bark and make a strong tea of it, and drink according as the patient may need. I have never known this to' fail — oftentimes when a violent flooding takes place, linen cloths wet in vinegar and water, and wrung out, and applied to the region of the belly, loins and thighs, and the same applications changed as they grow dry— and discontinued as the flooding ceases — but when all other means fail and have no effect, cold water dashed upon the patient's belly will stop the flooding immediately. Comfrey boiled in new milk, a little will stop them, and boiled in water will fetch them on:

NEGRO POISON.

The symptoms are often a devouring misery about the navel, and sometimes swells there, with a kind of griping pain, and sometimes a lax, and from that the pains will work upwards to the sides and across the ribs like the pleurisy, and under the shoulder blades; the bones will appear stiff and sore, the flesh will appear dead and sleepy; often break out in sores which is a favorable sign; the pulse is often high and hard, and often the breath short, and at other times the breath appears right; the lungs appear to be swelled. Whiskey or milk is pernicious to the complaint; there is oftentimes a swimming giddiness, the patient often craves what the poison is given in—the water is always of a high color, some have a good appetite, and

4

some have none. But let their appetite be as it will, the patients lose their flesh fast, and often the pains work from the top of the head to the end of toes.— When it is about to terminate in death, there is a deep sleeping ensues ; there is a cough that often follows the complaint, and sometimes a ratling in the lungs.— These are the most noted symptoms. And when the cough is bad, and the lungs are stopped, get a handful of horehound, the same of catnip, three or four roots of elecampane, boil these in half a gallon of water to a pint ; take out the herbs, and strain, then add half a pint of honey, the same of good apple vinegar, a spoonful of fresh butter the same of refined nitre, stew it down to half a pint, and give the patient a table spoonful every three or four hours, or as needful.— This medicine is to loosen the cough. The medicine necessary to remove the complaint, is—to get a handful of running brier roots, the same of sassafras bark, the same of the bark of the yellow poplar, the same of ginseng root, a gill of green plantain juice, and a handful of the twiggs of white ash tops, boil these to a decoction, and give the patient to drink often ; let their diet be light and cooling, not to eat hogmeat, sweet milk and pickle pork, nor heat your blood—beware of getting wet. Or you may take about three ounces of silk weed roots well cleansed, put them into a quart of spirits, drink of this two or three times a day—to take the dry roots and pulverize them in a mortar and sieve them—you may take a tea spoonful of these powders in a little honey, and drink warm water—this is as good a puke as nature can afford. Or get a handful of garlic, a gill of green plaintain juice, a table spoonful of brimstone, put these articles in a quart of rye whiskey, take of this morning and evening : this has cured many. Or fill a ten gallon pot with sour wood leaves, boil them well, take them out fill the pot again with water and the same kind of leaves, and boil them thoroughly—and then take out the leaves ; now you may fill the pot with wild cherry tree leaves, boil them in the same water by filling the pot with fresh water, boil out all the strength you can get, then take out the leaves, and add a handful of black snake roots to the same liquor and boil it well—and take out all the drugs—and add to this preparation a table spoonful of fine copperas—when it begins to thicken, add a spoonful of fine beat brimstone, and stew it down to a mass, and form it into pills, the size of a pea take one pill in the morning and two in the evening—while the patient is taking these pills he should keep from exposure of every kind and to refrain from eating hog meat and sweet milk.— But may be allowed to eat chickens, squirrels, beef, mutton, and to drink broths made from the same.— This medicine is also good for the Cachexy, Dropsy and to renew the blood.

THE WHITE SWELLING OF THE JOINTS.

This complant is often thought light of, but it is a growing evil ; the complaint is so well known that I need not describe but a few symptoms : It generally comes about the joints ; and seldom ever changes the color of the flesh, but rises to a head, and breaks, if not prevented, which affects the bone more and more, until it rises like a honey comb. But if this complaint is taken in time it is easily removed ; but if it gets the the mastery, it is not easily subdued; something like a small twig, which is easily bent when young, but afterwards becomes very stubborn. In the first, take a double handful of dogwood bark, the same of black haw bark, the same of ash bark, and when it is boiled well take out the barks, and put in a double handful ot mullin roots, and boil it down to a quart, and thicken it with meal, then let it get cool, and stir in it the white of three eggs, then spread the plaster on a cloth, and spread some honey on the plaster, end put it on the swelling, let this poultice stay there a day ; and take off that poultice, then boil cheerry tree leaves, black haw bark and dogwood bark, and white ass-smart; boil this well ; then take out the bark, then cut up some tobacco fine, and stew it well, then put in some apple vinegar, and thicken it the same way, put no honey on ; after that poultice comes off, give the patient a dose of salts ; let the poultice stay on twelve hours if possible ; their application will make the patient sick, but there will be no danger attending it, then when that comes off, give the patient a dose of salts or calomel and jalap during the time. If the swelling does not seem to abate, get the inside bark of white walnut, and the inside bark of the root, beat them fine, add a little strong vinegar, apply this to the white swelling. This will draw a blister like flies on any part of the body except the stomach. Then when you draw blisters, wash it with new milk, then put on bess-wax and tallow, or take some marsh willow roots, mullin, the tops and roots, boil them strong, take out the herbs, and then put in some burnt dirt out of the back wall, or a dirt oven, beat it fine ; put a little strong vinegar with it, stir it well together, then put this to the white swelling ; this is wonderful to draw it to a head or carry it away. Blistering on the swelling, and purgiug is the finest thing in nature ; or take the bark of the roots of marsh willow, and mullin roots and tops, then when they are boiled, take them out and put in some burnt dirt out of the back wall or dirt oven, beat it fine, and put in a little strong apple vinegar, and stir them well together ; then put this to the white swelling. This is a wonderful medicine to bring it to a head or carry it away ; and if it breaks, make some wet-fire and put in it. The wet-fire is made thus ; get a peck of ivy leaves, and boil them strong, then get a good quantity of ash bark, the insde, and put it in a pot, and put the pot over a hot fire until it burns to ashes, then soak the lye out of the ashes, and put the strength of the

leaves and the lve together, and boil it down to a pint;
and put this preparation in the place once or twice a
day, and let it stay on one hour and a half; then you
are to put in another salve ; the salve is to cleanse the
sore, and heal the inside, the salve is to be made thus :
"Take muscle shells, burn them well, and beat to a
powder, and let them soak in a little water, then take a
half pint of the water, and add to it half a pint of sweet
oil, stew them well, and put in the sore as above directed. Or make another kind of salve, (if it corrupts
and runs much,) that is made thus ; get a double
handful the root of dog wood bark, the same of yellow
sarsaparilla roots, the same of black oak bark, the
same of running briers roots, the same of wild cherry-
tree bark, the same of sassafras root, the bark, the
same of persimmon tree bark, get it off the north side
of the trees, then put them all together boil them half
a day add water occasionally, then take out barks and
strain it, then put the liquor back in the pot, boil it
down as thick as tar ; spread it on a cloth, and apply it
to the sore. This is a wonderful medicine to eat humors, sores and white swellings. If the white
welling becomes very painful, in any stage, take the
white of three eggs, mix them well with beat brimstone
and spread the poultice on soft leather, and put on
where the pain is : and if it is like to mortify, take some
wood dittany and beat it well, put in a little water to
make soft, and bind it to the swelling : or beat ground
ivy, and bind to it ; or take a handful of feathers, and
a roll of brimstone, and a little tar, put them in a pot,
on hot coals of fire, and hold the mortified place over
this (but keep the steam from your face ;) or get horehound, beat it well, and mix honey with it, and apply
to the place ; wood lime, dogwood bark, and white
walnut bark, boiled and thickened with rye meal, make
a poultice and bind to the place, &c. The following
makes a wonderful salve to carry away white swellings.
Take twelve eggs, and one pound of fresh butter, un-

washed, put these together and stew them moderately, add to this some rye meal stir it down to an ointment, keed this to anoint with: then get some oats, heat them, and put the same in a small bag, anoint with the oil, and put on the bag as hot as you can bear it, night and morning ; and when it begins to suage, or come to a head, apply a poultice made of swamp willows. This has cured many ; or put on eight or ten leeches once a day, and gentle vomits two or three times a week.— An electric may be used in every case when it can be done ; this remedy will frequently succeed. When appearances are unfavorable, bathe in salt and water often, or pump cold water on the knee, or part affected, half an hour. This seldom fails of curing pains in the joints. You may daily teem warm or cold water on the affected part, the warm water one day the cold water next, &c. I have given every necessary information relative to the treatment of this fatal diease &c.

THE HYSTERICS, &c.

Misses are sometimes subject to hysteric affections about the time of their first menstruation. This is an unfortunate circumstance, when ever it occurs, inasmuch as such will be liable to them for many years afterwards. A complete cure of this disease is seldom obtained; but there is some ground to hope for a recovery, if the proper remedies be employed on the first attack; or before it is deeply rooted in the system. This truly distressing complaint, puts on a great variety of shapes ; it is called protens of diseases, imitating almost every disorder to which the human body is subject. But I shall confine myself to the description of those symptoms which are most remarkable, the principal and discriminating marks are the following:—A peculiar kind of suffocation; this generally begins with a perception of a globe or ball, rolling round, seemingly among the bowels, and rising up to the stomach and throat, and there inducing strangling. This generally excites great alarm, with most excruciating fear of immediate death; consequently it will be attended with great paleness, and a profuse discharge of limpid urine; and unusual gurgling of the bowels, as if some little animal were there in actual motion; with wandering pains, constituting cholic of a peculiar kind; frequent efforts to vomit without any evacuation. This is sometimes mistaken for a symptom of inflammatory affection of the stomach, and their intestines; in this case there is always a great weakness of the stomach; a considerable degree of indigestion and anxiety, and sometimes a difficulty of breathing, with alternate flashings of heat and chilly sensation over different parts of the body; to those particular distinctions may he added alternate laughing and weeping, without any known or adequate cause; faintings, convulsions and palpitation, or fluttering of the heart; hysterical convulsions may be distinguished by the great fear of dying, which is peculiar to hysterics. For the cure, observe the following prescriptions: If the first attack of it, be the consequence of difficult or obstructed menstruation, let blood freely from the foot, and this the more certainly, if she was strong and healthy before the attack. If the sense of suffocation be violent, applying strong vinegar or spirits of harts-horn to her nose; bathe her feet in warm water; apply pretty severe friction to the region of her stomach, with a flesh brush, or flannel; and in some instances, a glyster of very cold water affords instant relief. When her health and spirits begin to decline, by no means be persuaded to confine her to her room, nor expect to restore her by heat or medicine only; instead of confinement, carry her abroad into agreeable company, turn her attention to some interesting employment, and let her diet be light and cooling. There are many causes for this complaint; according to the state of the system, I shall make three variations: The first is generally brought on by some exposure or accident. In this case, there will be a sensible fullness or increased motion of the blood, producing a swimming giddiness, a dull heavy pain of the head, which are increased by stooping down, a redness, fulness, with a sense of weight across the eyes; an aversion to motion; an unusual sense of weakness and heaviness of all the limbs; and sometimes a bleeding at the nose; a dead heavy misery across the small of the back. . Where these symptoms occur, let blood from the foot, ten or twelve ounces, repeated as occasion may require. Second, bathe her feet half an hour on going to bed. Third, then give a portion of calomel and aloes, three grains of each; syrup of some kind may be added so as to form it into a pill, or two, or so much as to make it of the consistence of honey; continue the bath, calomel and aloes, for three successive nights. If the disorder comes on suddenly, and she was healthy before, you may use the lancet the more; if she was delicate and feeble before the attack, use the vinegar or the spirits of harts-horn, and warm bath to the feet, &c. But if the obstruction of the menses be not the cause as above, according to circumstances, be cautious about letting blook. . For the radical cure in this last case, apply a blister to the stomach; use friction nearly all over the skin; give strong camomile tea to drink, wine, bark and steel dust, may be used; riding on horse-back, being in cheerful company and interesting engagements is beneficial to the afflicted patient. And in many instances there may be great benefit derived from the use of the following pill: that is to say—Take of asafœtida half an ounce, of Rusian castor one quarter of an ounce, and opium one quarter of an ounce, these ingredients are to be carefully beaten and mixed well together, and from this mass you must make two hundred pills of equal size; take three of these pills at night and two in the morning. If the patient be costive they may derive great advantage from the following composition: take aloes, one ounce, asafœtida half an ounce, the same of Rusian castor, and one quarter of an ounce of opium—mix these as the above, and form the same quantity of pills of equal size, and take in the same way, increasing or lessening the number according to the state of the bowels. The vitriolic either given from thirty to fifty drops, in a cup of some kind of drink, sometimes affords instant relief; when the suffocation is considerable and distressing, this article must be given speedily to prevent its loss by evaporation; and must not be opened too near a candle, because of its great readiness to take fire, &c. I have known the filings of gold taken night and morning in honey, to cure one that had been past work for three years; the dose may be about two or three grains. Or take beefs gall and put in rum, and drink as a bitter, it is a wonderful remedy in this case. And when the choking is bad, a tea spoonful of wheat flour, mixed in water and drank, will stop it; or chew orange peels and swallow the same.

THE BITE OF A SNAKE AND OTHER POISONOUS ANIMALS; HOW CURED.

If a person be bit by a snake, beat black ash leaves and bind to the wound as soon as possible, and make a tea of the bark; this will cure any snake bite; or give the patient a sweat of seneca snake root, over night and give him a tea spoonful of the juice of puccoon root in the morning. I have never known this medicine to fail, and there have been hundreds cured by it; or bind the liver and guts of the snake to the bite; or apply bruised garlic; or take a quantity of horehound, bruise it well in a mortar, and squeeze out the juice, likewise plantain in like manner, a table spoonful of each mixed together, and a table spoonful to be taken every hour for three hours, then every three hours till the infusion is done; and put the beaten herb to the bite—-or the juice of green plantain and new milk mixed together and drink, or if the patient be far spent, put a poultice of garlic to the bottom of the feet, or bind salt and tobacco to the bite, or take cucold bur leaves and bruise them, put in sweet milk, strain and drink the same.

SCROFULA, OR KINGS EVIL.

Scrofula consists in hard indolent tumors of the conglobate glands in various parts of the body; but particularly behind the ears, and under the chin, which after a time separates and degenerates into ulcers; from which, instead of pus, a white curdled matter, somewhat resembling the coagulum of milk, is discharged. The first appearance of the disease is most usually between the third and severth year of the childs age. But it may arise at any period between these and the age of puberty; after which it seldom makes its first attack. It most commonly affects children of a lax habit, with a smooth, soft, and fine skin, fair hair, rosy cheeks and a delicate complexion; but it is occasionally met with in those of a dark one. It likewise is apt to attack such children as show a disposition to rachitis, and marked by a protuberant forehead, enlarged joints, and a tumid abdomen. Scrofulous persons are often comely and rather distinguished for acuteness of understanding and precocity of genius. They are, however, seldom robust, or able to endure much fatigue without having their strength greatly exhausted, and their flesh much wasted; but when they once begin to regain these, their convalescense is usually rapid. Scrofula prevails most in those climates where the atmosphere is cold and humid, where seasons are variable and the weather unsteady. From latitude forty to sixty is the principal climate of the disease. A long continuance of inclement weather may increase any predisposition to Scrofula: and in persons already much predisposed to it, any uncommon, though temporary exposure to wet and cold, is sometimes an exciting cause of an immediate attack. Besides climate, and exposure to moist air and atmospherical vicissitude, every other circumstance which weakens the constitution, and impairs the general strength of the system, predisposes to Scrofula; thus breathing impure air unfit for respiration, and living upon food of an unwholesome and indigestible nature, which does not afford due nourishment to the body, favors an attack of Scrofula, by reducing the stiength of the system, and making the person weakly. The neglect of due personal cleanliness and of salutary exercise, indolence, inactivity, the want of warm clothing, confinement in cold damp habitations, &c., may all be regarded as so many exciting causes, and satifactorily account for the prevalence of disease among children employed in large manufactories, as at Manchester, &c. Scrofula is by no means a contagious disease, but beyond all doubt is of an hereditary nature, and is often entailed by parents on their children. The patient it is true is not born with the disease, but only with a greater aptitude to receive certain morbid impressions, which may bring the latent disposition into action. There are indeed some practitioners who wholly deny that this or any other disease can be acquired by an hereditary right; but that a peculiar temperament of the body, bias, or predisposition in the constitution to some diseases, may extend from both Father and Mother to their offspring, is, I think, very clearly proved; for example, we very frequently meet with gout in young persons of both sexes, who could never have brought it on by intemperance, sensuality or improper diet, but must have acquired the predisposition to it in this way. A remarkable circumstance attending the transmission of scrofula, is, that although it is an hereditary disease, it does occasionally pass over one generation and appear again in the next, so that the Grandfather and Grandson, (the first and third generations,) shall both be scrofulous, while the intermediate one which holds the more intimate relation of Father and son, and connects the two others together, shall be exempted from any attack of the disease. The attacks of scrofula seem much affected or influenced by the periods of the seasons. They begin usually some time in the winter and spring, and often disappear; or are greatly amended in summer and autumn. The first appearance of the disorder is commonly in that of small oval or spherical tumors under the skin, unattended by any pain or discoloration, these appear in general, upon sides of the neck, or below the ear, or under the chin; but in some cases, the joints of the elbows, ancles, or those of the fingers and toes, are the parts first affected. In these instances we do not, however, find moveable swellings, but on the contrary, a tumor almost uniformly surrounding the joint, and interrupting its motion. After some length of time, the tumors become larger and more fixed, the skin which covers them acquires a purple or livid color, and being much inflamed, they at least separate and break into little holes, from which at first a matter somewhat puriform oozes out; but this changes by degrees into a kind of viscid serous discharge much intermixed with small pieces of a white substance, resembling the curd of milk. In the treatment of this disorder, there is several things very necessary to be noticed, as the general symptoms have been accurately laid down, there will be no difficulty of forming a correct idea of the disease. If in case this disorder should be taken in time there will be but little difficulty of performing a cure,

but where it has been of long standing ,it is generally
more obstinate. Where the glands of the neck appear
to be affected, and somewhat swelled; it is necessary
it should be set running on each side of the neck, this
may be,done by applying a small portion of nitric acid
or aquafortis. Those places should be kept running by
the use of salves, poultices, &c., until the swelling entirely leaves the neck, at the same time while pursuing
this course, the patient should take the following preparation — Get a peck of the inside bark of the root of
dogwood, the same of black oak, the same of the roots
of sumac, the same of wild cherrytree bark, this you
will boil in ten gallons of water down to two, this liquid should then be strained ; to this preparation there
should be added, one quart of Maderia Wine, twenty
grains of tartar emetic, two pounds of sugar, twenty
grains of refined nitre, this should all be completely
dissolved together, it is then fit for use, the patient
should take a table spoonful three times per day, the
diet should be very limited while using this medicine,
the patient should take half a table spoonful of the
cream of tartar every fourth day dissolved in a little
cold water; bleeding is also necessary at times ; if in
case the eyes are affected, there should be a blister
drawn on the back of the neck, and be kept running
for some length of time, the eyes should be frequently
bathed in a weak solution of the sugar of lead. If in
case the glands under the arm should become affected,
that is swetted, they should be well bathed every night
and morning with the following ointment: take four
ounces of the oil of sassafras or pennyroyal, the same
of the spirits of turpentine, two ounces of sulphuric
ether, one ounce of laudanum, mix this well together,
it is then fit for use. This course of treatment should
be well pursued, until every symptom disappear — it is
then necessary that the system should be strengthened
by mild tonics, such as barks, quinine, and all strengthening medicines — if in case the lungs should become

debilitated, the preparations under the head "Pulmonary
Consumption" should be strictly attended to.

    Afflicted patients with this disease,
    Have often come to me for ease;
    [Tho' much distressed have been their case,
    I have never failed in curing them.]
    I have never fail'd in curing all,
    Who to me have made a call.

THE DISEASE OF CHILDREN, OR VOMITING.

When what has been taken is returned crude and
unaltared, it may be suspected to arise from over-feed-
ing, and to require nothing more than temperance for
its cure. Vomiting, however, is often an attendant on
other complaints, as sometimes of itself constitutes an
original disease. Where there is a vomiting of digested food, it will be right to change the mode of diet, or
to open the body by some gentle aperient. If these
means do not answer, and the vomiting continues, it
will be proper to clear the stomach by a gentle emetic,
afterwards giving the saline medicine in an effervesing
state, with a drop or two of the tincture of opium.
We may at the some time apply a blister over the region of the stomach, or rub it well with an anodyne
liniment.

SUSPENDED ANIMATION AND RESUSCITATION.

In consequence of drowning, and also of suffocation
and strangulation, a considerable check is often given to
the principle of life, without wholly extinguishing it.—
When it happens from the first of these causes, the circulation becomes gradually more feeble and slow, and
much anxiety is felt about the precordia ; to relieve

which, the person atttempts to rise to the surface of the water : he then discharges a quantity of air from the lungs, and receives into them a very small portion of water, when he again sinks. After struggling in this manner for some short time, convulsive spasms arises, the organs of respiration ceases to act, and he at last expires ; soon after which the skin becomes of a purple or blue cast, particularly about the face and neck, and the body sinks. It has been supposed, and the opinion is indeed still very general among the common people, that in the act of drowning, the wates enters the lungs and completely fills them. Experience, however, has shown, that unless the body lies so long in the water, as to have its living principle entirely destroyed, the quantity of fluid present in the lungs is inconsiderable ; for upon drowning kittens, puppies, &c, in ink, other colored liquors, and afterwards examining the viscera, it has been observed that very little of the colored liquor has gained admittance to them. The circumstance may be readily accounted for by recollecting that the muscles which form the opening into the trachea are exquisitely sensible, and contract violently upon the least irritation, as we frequently experience when any part of the food or drink happens to come in contact with them. When a young person dies from suffocation, the symptoms are nearly the same as in apoplexy. The phenomena which attend on strangulation are, convulsive paroxysms superadded to the apoplectic symptoms.— Livid and dark brown spots on the face, with great rigdity coldness of the body, a glassy appearance of the eyes and a flacid state of the skin, denote a perfect extinction of life ; but the only certain sign is actual putrefaction ; and therefore, in every case where this symptom is not present, and where we are acquainted with the length of time the body may have been under water, every possible means shouid be employed immediately upon its being found for restoring it to life,

as the noble machine may be stopped and the spring
nevertheless still retain, in some degree, its elastic vig-
or. Dissections of those who have died by drowning,
show that an accumulation of blood in the venous system, forms the great morbid change which takes place
in accidents of this nature. The lungs are in a stae of
collapse, and the accumulation of blood is confined to
the venacave, the heart, and the parts of the venous
system. In some cases the stomach is found to contain a small quantity of water ; in others, none is to be
perceived. From the muscles of the trachea having
lost the principle of life, upon which, the power of muscular contraction depends they become relaxed, the water enters the wind pipe. In all instances, the external
surface of the brain appears of a highly florid color,
without any great distention of vessels or marks of effusion. It has been supposed however, by many, that
persons who die by drowning suffer from the intervention of apoplexy. After a recovery from apoplexy, the
person is generally paralytic, whereas, no such event
following the recovery from a suspension of life by drown
ing, the proximate cause appears to be the stoppage of
air to the lungs. The following are the means to be employed for the recovery of persons recently drowned. As
soon as the body is taken out of the water it is to be
speedily conveyed in men's arms, or be placed upon
a door, or in a cart upon straw. If the distance is considerable, to the nearest house, where it is quickly to be
stripped of the wet clothes ; to be wiped perfectly dry ;
and then to be laid btween warm blankets, spread upon
a mattress or low table, and on the right side in prefer-
ence to the left. In order that the passage of the
blood from the heart may be favored by the position
The head is at the same to be covered with a woolen
cap, being properly elevated with pillows, and bags
filled with warm sand, or bricks heated and wrapped in
flannel, are to be applied to the feet. The doors and
windows of the apartment are to be thrown open, in

order that the cool air may be freely admitted, ard no persons but such as are necessary to give due assistance, should be allowed to enter.

Having taken these steps, we should next endeavor to expand the lungs, and make them, if possible, reassume their office. When not furnished with a flexible tube made of elastic gum, and of a sufficient length or with the bellows invented for this express purpose (which is of such a construction, that, by one action, fresh air is thrown into the lungs, and by another it is thrown out again, so as to imitate or produce artificial breathing,) we must be content with blowing in air by means of a common pair; or by inserting a pipe into one nostril, compressing the other, shutting the person's mouth at the same time, and then blowing through the pipe with a considerable degree of force. By any of these means we may be enabled to inflate the lungs.—At the same time that the lungs are inflated, we should rub every part of the body with warm flannel cloths.—On all occasions it will be the best way to divide the assistants into two sets; the one being employed in endeavoring to restore the heat of the body; the other, in instituting an artificial breathing in the manner Just pointed out.

Should the frictions not be attended with any effect, we ought to apply flannel cloths, wrung out in very hot water, over the heart and thorax, or we may put the person in a warm bath. A high degree of heat will not be necessary; a moderate degree will be sufficient. If the weather be under the freezing point, and the body, when stripped, feels cool, and nearly in the same condition with one that is frozen, it will be necessary at first, to rub it well with snow, or wash it with cold water, the sudden application of heat in such cases having been found very pernicious. In a short time, however, warmth must be gradually applied. To assist in rousing the vital principle, it has been customary to

5

apply various stimulating matters, such as common salt, and rectified and also volatile spirits, to different parts of the body; but, as the skin looses its sensibility in pioportion as it is deprived of heat, and does not recover it again until the natural degree of warmth be restored, it is obvious, that previous to the restoration of heat, all such applications are useless. Rectified spirits evaporate fast, and thereby, instead of iecreasing warmth, as they are expected to do, carry off a part of the heat from the body. Volatile spirits are liable to the same objections, and are, besides, distressing to the eyes of the assistants. Common salt quickly frets the skin, and has, in some cases, produced sores which were difficult to heal after recovery. When there is reason to think the skin has, in some degree, recovered its sensibility, the wrists, ancles, temples, and parts over the stomach and heart, may be rubbed with a little of the linimentum ammoniac carbonatis, or (the tincture of worm-wood.) In a case of suspended animation, it may be necessary to stimulate the stomach and intestines, the stomach may be stimulated with a small portion of the tincture of gum myrrh, the latter may be done by an injection of strong senna tea combined with a little paragoric. When the patient is so far recovered as to be able to swallow, he should be put into a warm bed with his head and shoulders properly elevated with pillows, warm wines, weak todies, should be given in moderate quantities, the feet and legs should be completely bound over with warm flannels wrung out in hot vinegar, this course should be pursued until relief is obtained

THE VENEREAL DISEASE.

This is a complaint that goes to and fro through the land. There are many unfortunate, poor unhappy persons that for fear of disgrace, endure pain both in body and mind, rather than go to a doctor at first. Some friend or secret keeper replies he has got a cure. Well, the method is tried; but this remedy only removes the symptoms for a space, which corrupts the blood, and flings the patient in a worse situation, which is often incurable. The innocent can take the effects of this complaint as well as the guilty — infants nurses, mid-wives, and women by guilty husbands. If you are innocently taken in, you are excusable. Though he that has taken the blaze on the other hand, is condemned by Pauls' ministerial word, for he says, it is better to marry than to burn; and generally when the flame takes place, there is a discharge of matter, which makes its appearance within eight or ten days after the infection has been received, and some within two or three days, according to what state the blood is in when you take it, and with some not under four or five weeks; but the patient often feels an itching with a small degree of pain in the testicles, and sometimes there runs a yellow thin water which stains, and with some it is white with a violent burning when they make water: and it comes sometimes with a degree of heat, and there is often a redness. If the disorder is not checked, the symptoms will increase; the disorder rises higher and higher in the penis, and the longer it runs the worse the patient dreads to make water, but wants to be always at it, until it will come by drops, in this complaint; tho' there is a disorder in women that one might be mistaken in, that is, when the womb is affected, and there comes a whitish matter and sometimes a kind of greenish color, and with some their terms are discharged in this way. Now regard should be had to eating and drinking, no strong drink, nor salted nor smoaked meats, nor heat your blood, and do not season what you eat too high; drink cooling teas, balm, ground ivy, sink-field, mallad, &c., in the first place take a good dose of salts, or calomel and jalap, syringe with blue stone and apple brandy, two or three times a day; and you may take of may apple, root; make it thus:

take one handful of may apple roots, and put the same in a pot and add a quart of water, boil them very strong, take a table spoonful inwardly, and if this does not operate, you should take another, and so on until it does work; then take a handful of sarsaparilla, and wild cherry tree bark, the high black berry brier roots, the bark of the roots of white sumac, a handful of dogwood bark, half a handful of red oak bark, a handful of the bark of yellow poplar roots, a double handful of pine tops, boil these altogether until they are strong; take of this three or four times a day, and if ulcers or sores arises, or blubbers, apply red precipitate dissolved in old whiskey to wash with; until, and after taking this, purge with salts, and bleed, &c.—or take a handful of dogwood bark, the same of running brier roots, the same of yellow poplar bark, the same of rattle root, the same of sumac, add a quart of water for each handful, boil it strong, drink of this often and let your diet be light; keep from hog meat, salted fish, or smoked meats; take care of taking cold, wet, or heating your blood. You may drink cooling tea; or take a handful of yellow poplar bark, the same of sumac root, the same of dogwood bark, the same of yellow sarsaparilla roots, the same of sassafras bark, boil these well and drink it for your constant drink; make use of flaxseed and comfrey teas when going to bed.

INFLAMMATION OF THE EYES, OR SORE EYES.

Sore eyes are of two kinds that which affects the coats of the balls of the eye, &c.—that which affects the eyelids only. The causes inducing inflammation are external violence, wounds, particles of dust, sand, &c., or the hairs of the eye lids inverted, too much light, or strong light too long continued; sitting up at night before a fire, riding in snow, particularly when it falls early or late in the season, writing or reading too much at night, too long accurately inspecting very minute objects, frequent intoxication, sharp matter, such as tobacco, &c., received into the eyes ; sympathy sore eyes, frequently taken by looking at others in the same condition, and is the effect of an active imagination. General fever sometimes produces this disease. ' The remedies are as follows — bleeding, when there is general fever, copious bleeding from the arm will be necessary ; if no general fever present, cupping the temples and scarifying the inside of the eye lids. Purges may be more or less violent, according to the violence of the disease. Blisters should be applied to the neck and behind the ears, and to the temples. Certain washes ; these must be mild or sharp, according to the stage of the disease. In most instances when inflammation of the eyes first appears, cold water, milk and water, or mild lead water will be proper ; the lead water should be made into a poultice and applied to the eye affected, first covering it with a bit of cambric or muslin. In the last stages of this disease, the eyes may be washed with the following solution ; take two drachms of white vitriol, and forty grains of the sugar of lead, and add these to a gill of spring water — If these articles be not convenient you may take weak spirits and water, Maderia wine and water, salt and water, or a decoction of oak bark and leaves not too strong. In curing this disease, the patient should not be exposed to the light, and all spirituous liquors must be carefully avoided. When there are particles of dust, or the like in the eye, it may sometimes be washed out with clean water ; if an inverted hair be the cause it must be plucked out. If the disease should be of long standing and obstinate setons, and issues will be proper. The eyes should be washed with salt petre water, then with breast milk or honey and copperas mixed well together ; or take a table spoonful of white copperas, the same of salt, put these to a quart of water, and boil it down to a pint, then let it settle, pour it off and let it settle, and boil it down to a half pint, keep this to wash any humor in the eyes; take angelica, and boil it in water, then mix it in new milk, and wash the eyes, and at night bind rotten apples to them when going to bed; or take half an ounce of lapis calaminarlis powdered into a half pint of French white wine, and as much white rose water, put a drop or two in the corner of the eye, this has cured some that have been nearly blind; or take six ounces of rectified spirits of wine, dissolve it in one drachm of camphor, then add two handfulls of dried elder flowers and when you wash your eyes, wash your forehead also.

A GENERAL DESCRIPTION OF WORMS IN CHILDREN

The symptoms pointing out the presence of worms are various, and are the following to-wit: Grinding of the teeth, starting in sleep, a dry cough bringing up a frothy spittle, sighing, and suffocating manner of breathing, pain in the side, hiccough, heart burn, vomiting, lax, sudden urgings to go to stool, costiveness, slimy stools, night sweats, sour breath, flushing of one cheek, itching of the nose, an excessive appetite, lying much on the belly, a swelling of the partition of the nose and of the upper lip, the actual voiding of more or less worms, a wasting away of the limbs and the whole body, jaundice, head-ache, deadly snoring in sleep, convulsions, &c., &c. Our first care should be to prevent the dangerous effects of worms; and there are various articles of food, which will answer this intention: "nature," says Dr. Bush, in his medical enquiries, "has wisely guarded children against the morbid effects of worms, by implanting in them an early appetite for common salt, ripe fruits, and saccharine substances," all of which appear to be among the most speedy and effectual poisons for worms.— Ever since I observed the effects of sugar, and other sweet substances upon worms, I have recommended the liberal use of all of them in the diet of children, with the happiest effects. The remedies proper for the removal of worms are common salts; this may be given in doses of thirty grains, upon an empty stomach in the morning, and is an excellent remedy. Sugar or molasses in large quantities, so that they may pass out of the stomach, without undergoing any material change from digestion; in small quantities they will destroy worms in the stomach only. The pressed juice of onions and garlic are said to be considerably efficacious against the excess of worms. Gun-powder, a tea spoonful to be given in the morning, upon an empty stomach:—Carolina pink root: If this article be properly used, it is a certain remedy; about half an ounce may be gently stewed in half a pint of water, till its strength be properly extracted; and then let the decoction be strained and well sweetened with sugar or molasses, and give one fourth of it every two or three hours, to a child of four or five years old. I have generally thought it best to add to each dose, about one eighth of an ounce of manna. The importance of this addition will appear when it is remarked, that the pink root is poisonous, and if given in too large quantities, kills the child to whom it is given. Aloes, four to six grains; Rhubarb, eight to fifteen grains; Jesuits bark, bears-foot, worm-seed; these are all said to be medicines for worms: Calomel is a safe medicine, whether given by itself or combined with jalap. It is most effectual, however, when given in large doses; from four to eight grains, might be given to a child of four or six years old. But of all the medicines that I have administered, says Dr. Bush, I know of none more safe and certain than the simple preparation of iron, whether it be given in the form of steel filings, or of the rust of iron; if ever they fail of success, it is because they are given in too small doses—I generally prescribe from five to thirty grains every morning, for children be-

tween one and ten years old. I have been taught by
an experienced practitioner, that this remedy cured him
of a tape worm. The common prescribed dose is from
two drachms to half an ounce, every morning, for three
or four days—he took this not only with safety but
with success. I generally give it in honey, or take of
alum the size of a bean, and beat it fine, and mix with
honey for three or four days, this is also good, and may
be given without endangering the life of the child.

THE PUTRID SORE THROAT, &c.

This disease generally appears in autumn; and children are more subject to it than grown persons. It
generally follows moist, wet and hazy weather. The
principal symptoms attending it are great weakness,
slight eruption, weak, a quick pulse, and ulcers in the
throat. Delirium, especially at night; diarrhœa, inflamed and watery eyes, a flat and rattling voice, the
ulcers and sloughs in the throat are of a whitish ash
color, and the breath of the patient is very offensive to
the smell. The remedies are pukes, say ipecacuanha, ten
grains, and calomel four grains: to be taken together,
as a dose for a child of eight or ten years old; bark,
wine and cordial aliment; the bark should be given in
substance, but if that be impracticable, a decoction
may be substituted; Port wine should be preferred; if
wine cannot be had, a decoction of Virginia snake root,
is a tolerable substitute, chicken broth is the best diet,
and should be used as early as possible, in the disease;
blisters should be applied to the neck and throat; but
blisters drawn in this disease, should never be dressed
with colewort leaves; some kind of mild ointment
spread on a piece of fine linen, should be preferred for
this purpose: knead together, oil five parts, and bees-
wax one part; the mouth and throat should be washed
with barley water, or very thin gruel, to which should

be added a little vinegar and honey, and if convenient, a portion of the tincture of myrrh, might be added to half an ounce of the gruel, &c., or if the myrrh cannot be had, as much calomel might be added instead of it, as may be sufficient to turn it of a whitish color. I have found great benefit from frequently washing the mouth and throat well with the following mixture:— Take saft petre half an ounce, and borax one quarter of an ounce; the whole to be dissolved in one pint of water, and sweetened with honey. I have used it successfully in a number of cases, without any other topical application. The steams of vinegar and myrrh received into the throat by the help of a funnel, are sometimes beneficial. I have done wonders by this machine; that is to get, a handful of comfrey, the same of elecampane, boil this well in fresh spring water, then take out the roots, and put in a quart of hard apple cider and a pint of honey and receive the steam in the mouth with a funnel or coffee-pot, and bind a slice of wheat bread wet in brandy on the top of the head; and make a plaster of tallow and bind to the throat ;— this remedy is wonderful; this plaster put to the throat will take up the palate of the mouth, when it is down ; and tie the middle curl of the top of the head, will do the same ; or black pepper laid on the top of the point of a case knife, and put to the palate, will fetch it back.

PUERPERAL OR CHILD BED FEVER.

The puerperal fever comes on gradually, commencing in about twenty hours after delivery, and sometimes it is three or four weeks. Weak and delicate women, especially those accustomed to living a genteel life, are most subject to it. It begins with a chill, and the symptoms attending it are nausea, pain in the

head, loss of strength, restlessness : the skin is sometimes dry, at other timés partially or unusually moist;
the tongue is dry, covered with a black crust; the
pulse raises, being sometimes weak and small, then full
and hard ; wandering pains are felt in the abdomen —
at times they attack the sides, resembling the pleurisy ;
in some cases they extend to the shoulders, then descend to the bladder and lower intestines : the pain
becomes so accute in some instances, that the patient
cannot bear the least water on them ; the face has a
sorrowful appearance, and every word and action will
more or less express the sufferings of the patient; at
times the abdomen swells considerably ; pain is felt in
the small of the back ; the legs and feet swell ; at
length the breathing becomes difficult ; vomiting and
diarrhoea isometimes takes place ; the lochia are sometimes suppressed, at other times they continue throughout the disease ; when the inflammation is confined to
the uterus, this is a very favorable circumstance ; the
urine is generally very scanty and unfrequent ; turbid
spots appear on the joints, and sometimes on the face ;
although the appearances vary in difficult patients, yet
by the catalogue of symptoms this fever may be known,
On the first attack, the patient should be bled according to her strength and the violence of the attack, then
a mild vomit of fifteen grains of ipecacuanha with one
grain of tartarised antimony, should be given, worked
off with warm water.   Should there be any cramping
or pain in the stomach while vomiting, take ten drops
of laudanum, and drink freely of strong senna tea and
opiate at night, glysters fermentations and opening
drops of senna, manna, and cream of tartar combined
may daily be used until relieved.   If there be frequent
or voluntary stools, we must be cautious not to administer any thing which may do injury—in such cases,
glysters of chicken water, or flour and water boiled to
a proper consistency, or flax seed tea, ought to be
often repeated.   It requires some skill to determine

the propriety of correcting this diarrhœa, if however, it becomes necessary, through the debility of the patient to check it, an infusion of camomile flowers may be used with addition of a few drops of laudanum— should a hiccoughing come on, take the sweet spirits of nitre half an ounce, water half a pint, half an ounce of loaf sugar; of this mixture, give two table spoonfuls every three or four hours, ihe patient should breathe pure air, strict regard should be had to the cleanliness, and silence should be carefully observed, mild tonics of various kinds may be given in small doses, in this important case it is necessary to call in a physician, if one should be convenient, and not depend too much on old women, with their strong teas, hot rocks, &c.

ASIATIC CHOLERA.

The leading features of cholera and its pathological relation to diarrhœa have been in instances pointed out from the earliest times, it has been acknowledged as one of the most dangerous diseases to which the human body is subject, but the extreme malignity of which it is susceptible was never thoroughly known until these few years when it has been seen to spread with uncontrolable violence. Cholera makes its attacks in almost all cases suddenly and unexpectedly, it commences with nausea unremited and bile and vomiting, severe griping pains of the bowels, and generally puring, the matter rejected consisting partially if not principally of bile, it is attended with great thirst, a coated tongue, a small frequent and feeble pulse a cold skin, and buried irregular respiration, the prostration of strength which accompanies it and the rapidity with which it advances gives to this disease a peculiar character and renders it one of very urgent danger, in many cases when un checked it proceeds so rapidly that in a ·few hours the patient is brought into a state of considerable risk, cramps of the legs, extending to the thighs, abdominal muscles and diaphragm combine with the incessant vomiting and purging, to exhaust the patient's strength and if relief be not speedily obtained are followed by coldness of the extremeties and of the whole skin extreme restlessness, clamy sweat hickup and death, in general there is no pain of the abdomen on pressure and little or no delirium the patient dying from exhaustion of nervous power. Cholera is not usually attended by febrile symptoms, unless indeed we acknowledge that to be a febrile state which the ancienis call Lyperia, where the inward parts burn, and the skin feels cold.— In this country cholera has proved fatal in six hours, it seldom lasts longer than three or four days, it occurs principally in the months of July and August and appears to be altogether dependent upon some peculiar influence of a heated atmosphere, on the symptom a violence of the disease is almost always proportioned to the heat of the preceeding summer.

I have laid down a few of the general symptoms of this upleasant disease, I shall now endeavor to give my mode of treatment, having had a very extensive practice in cases of cholera in Kentucky, when it raged with such uncontrolable violence in that state ; first when their appears to be a derangement of the stomach and bowels, the patient complaining of severe misery either in the bowels or stomach, give twenty grains of pulverised mandrake (or mayapple root,) combined with one grain of opium, three of camphor, and four of cayene peper, three drops of the oil of croton, this should be mixed in a little water and sugar, this medicine will operate severely on the bowels, in about one hour after it is taken, when it begins to operate, the patient should drink waim teas, soup, &c., if in case this does not appear to give immediate relief, heavy portions of blood should be taken from the arm and the patient well bathed in warm water, and another dose of

the above prescription given as before, laudanum may
be given in small quantities, frequently stimulating liquors may be freely used, but it is sometimes the case
and indeed frequently, that persons are attacked ap-
pearently at once with cholera, when this is the case, it is
very probable that in a half hour the patient is completely
cramped through the whole extremity ; in this stage you
will discover large drops of cold clamy sweat on the face,
the feet cold, the eyes sunk the countenace greatly changed, where this is the case give a tea spoonful of the oil of
black mustard seed, in a little honey combined with a
hundred drops of the tincture of opium, this medicine
will have the tendency of throwing the blood throug
the whole extremities, whenever the regular circula-
tions take place give a vomit of tartar emetic or some
other emetic, immediately, in two hours after you give
the vomit, give ten drops of the oil of croton, this should
be repeated every four hours if necessary ; the patent
should be well rubbed in warm liquors, keep warm in
his bed, mild tonics may also be given freely, many other
things could be recommended as it is frequently the
case that it would be inconvenient for the people of
the country to get them, the best plan is when you ap-
prehend danger send for the best physician you can
get, for unless immediate relief can be had, death is the
consequence.

HEPATITIS, OR CHRONIC INFLAMMATION OF THE LIVER.

Pyrexia, tension, and pain of the right hypocondrium, often pungent as in pleuritis, but sometimes dull,
pain in the clavicle and top of the right shoulder, uneasy lying on the left side, difficult respiration, dry
cough and vomiting, are the characteristics of the hepatitis ; very frequently there is some degree of jaundice.
Hepatitis has generally been considered of two kinds ;

the one acute, the other chronic; the former shewing
the essential character of genuine inflammation: the
latter exhibiting symptoms of a less violence as to their
inflammatory tendency, but an enlargement and hardness of the liver with an obtuse pain.   Besides the
causes producing other inflammation, such as the application of cold, external injuries from contusions, blows,
&c., this disease may be occasioned by violent exercise,
by intense summer heats, by long continued intermittent and remittent fever, by high living, and an inter-
perate use of vinous and spirituous liquors, but more
particularly the latter, and by various solid concritions
in the substance of the liver.   Derangement of the digestive organs, suppressed secretions, inflammations,
compression, fevers and mental solicitude, are very general causes of obstructions and diseases of the liver.
The acute species of Hepatitis comes on with a sense
of chillness, preceding pain in the hypocondrium, sometimes dull, sometimes sharp, extending up to the clavicle and shoulder of that side most usually, which is
much increased by pressing upon the part, and is accompanied with a cough, oppression of breathing, and
difficulty of lying except on the side affected ; together
with nausea and sickness and often with a vomiting of
bilious matter; the intestines are generally inactive,
and the stools show a deficiency of biliary secretion, or
at least of any intermixture of it with them : the urine
is of a deep saffroon color, and small in quantity; there
is loss of appetite, great thirst, and costiveness, with a
strong, hard, and frequent pulse, of from ninety to one
hundred in a minute and sometimes intermitting: the
skin is dry and hot at the same time, and the tongue
covered with a white and sometimes a yellowish fur; and
when the disease has continued for some days, the skin
and eyes become tinged of a deep yellow, particularly
when the inflammation is produced by calculi in the
parenchyma of the liver.   In hepatitis, as well as in
other diseases we do not always find the symptoms of

the same degree of violence as they are described in
the definition; thus in some cases the fever is severe,
in others it is scarcely perceptible; in some instances
the pain is very acute and violent; in others collections
of pus have been found after death, when no pain was
felt. When the pain is seated deep in the substance
of the liver, as that possesses little sensibility, the pain
is usually obtuse, but when the surface is affected, it
is acute, and apt to spread to the diaphragm and lungs,
producing cough. What constitutes great difficulty in
managing hepatitis is, that in many cases the symptoms which are primary and indicative of inflammatory
affection, are but very slightly, marked, even when it
is in such a degree as to run with readiness into suppur-
ation, and particularly in the east and west Indies.
The pain in the sides is not constant or acute, the patient himself takes little notice of it, and when question-
ed concerning it, he only tells you perhaps, that he has
felt at times slight pains about the pit of the stomach, or
in the right side. It is only by observing the secondary symptoms, such as, a diarrhœa, or short dry cough
and pain felt at the top of the shoulder, or that there
is a degree of fullness or tenderness on pressing on the
organ a little hard, with some yellowless of the eyes
and countenance, that the true state and nature of the
disorder is to be ascertained in such cases. During the
inflammatory stage of the acute hepatitis, it will be proper to adapt bleeding particularly where the pain appears to be acute, the regular functions of the stomach
should be brought into complete action and the inflammation should be allayed as much a possible, as the
blood is much disordered in this case with a general
debility of the whole system, it will be very necessary
that the blood should be purified and brought into a
proper state, this may be done by using the liquid, described in the case of dyspepsia, it should be taken also
in the same way as there directed; blistering on the
back of the neck and pit of the stomach is also neces-

sary. Ten grains of rhubarb, three of mandrake, five of calomel well mixed together in a little honey, should be taken every other night, this should be pursued for several times in succession, until it produces some action on the saliva glands, also the bowels, the diet should be gruel, broth, &c. As a tonic the compound of spikenard, as directed in the materia medica, should be strictly taken. Two ounces of charcoal, the same of magencia, should be well pulverised together, and half a table spoonful taken every morning in a little sweet milk. A tincture of aloes, assafœdita, horsemint, Indian turnip, should be used freely as a tonic. The tincture of quinine, angelica, may also be used at times. There is but little danger attending this disease if taken in time; when you discover a shifting pain in the stomach, in the shoulders, back of the neck, do not think this a mere nothing, but endeavor to attend to the means immediately which are prescribed. Thereby, the patient may save trouble, pain and probably death. In the treatment of the chronic inflammation of the liver, the first thing necessary, is, the liver should be cleared of that torpid mucus and bile that is there collected this may be done by using the following powder: take of gum guiacum three ounces, of mandrake two ounces, of aloes half an ounce, pulverize these well together to a complete powder, and take half a table spoonful every third night in the white of an egg. This powder will act very powerfully upon the liver, will work off that slimy mucus that is there collected in the deranged state of the blood. The tincture of wormwood as described in the materia medica, should be taken, from twenty-five to fifty drops four or five times a day in a little water. Wine, barks, and ginger, mixed well together should also be taken, half a table spoonful two or three times a day. Ten drops of the tincture of lobelia should be taken every morning at sunrise, and should the bowels become rather loose, a few drops of laudanum or a small pill of kino may be taken;

the diet should be nothing but coarse corn bread and butterless-milk, rye mush, Irish potatoes, but not a particle of grease at any time should be used. I have endeavored to recommend such means as the people can get, and which are efficacious in this disorder, and if strictly attended to will have the desired effect.

PALPITATIO, OR PALPITATION.

This disease consists in a vehement and irregular motion of the heart, and is induced by organic affections ; a morbid enlargement of the heart itself, or of the large vessels, a diminution of the cavities of the ventricles, from inflammation or other causes, polypiosification of the aorta or other vessels, plethora, debility or mobility of the system, mal-conformation of the thorax, and many of the causes inducing syncope.

During the attack, the motion of the heart is performed with more rapidity, and generally with more force than usual, which is not only to be felt with the hand, but may be often perceived by the eye, and in some instances even heard ; there is frequently, dyspnœa, a purplish hue of the lips and cheeks, and a great variety of anxious and painful sensations. In some instances the complaint has terminated in death, but in many others it is merely symptomatic of hysteria, and other nervous disorders. As the disease, however, arises from an organic affection of the heart itself in many instances, or of the arota, or other large vessels connected with it, all that may be in our power in such cases will be to caution the patient against exposing herself, or himself, to such circumstances as may increase the action of the sanquiferious system, particularly fits of passion, sudden surprise, violent exercise

6

or great exertions of the body. In the treatment of this disease it should be our study if possible to find out the exciting causes, if it arise from plethora, bleeding with purgatives, and the rest of the antiphlogistic course should be adopted, if from debility take two ounces of green plantain, the same of the nside bark of cherry tree, the same of birch tree bark, boil these well together in half a gallon of vinegar down to one pint, after it is strained add one gill of honey, two grains of the flour of sulphur, three grains of refined nitre, of this the patient should take a table spoonful three times a day. If it should arise from any general debility of the nerves, a compound tincture of rue, horsmint, tanzy, should be used as described, that is, take thirty drops of either of the tinctures in a little water, at the same time keep the bowels moderately open, &c.

THE PILES·

Many persons are subject to this distressing complaint, both male and female are subject to it. This disorder by whatever means, the disposition to the Piles is formed, it generally is most troublesome in females in the last months of pregnancy, than at other times. If the attack be of a moderate kind, a gentle dose of the cream of tartar, and flour of sulphur combined, will afford considerable relief. Cold applications of any kind as of cloth wet in cold water, or spirits and water would answer the purpose. Also the following ontment :—Take the yolk of an egg, tincture of opium, or laudanum, three tea spoonfuls, neats foot oil or any other, one table spoonful to be mixed and applied; let the tincture and the yolk of the egg be first mixed together, and afterwards the oil may be added. This ointment gives relief when disposed, to itch ; if they produce outwards. press them between the thumb and

finger, and at the same time anoint and put them up
carefully. Those subject to this complaint ought to lie
down upon their backs for a few minutes after every
stool. I have known this precaution to do much towards preventing their return when once removed.—
I am told an ointment made of the oak ball powdered
and stewed in hogs lard, is a valuable remedy, and
there is no reason to doubt its value. Steep butterfly
root, and drink as a tea, is a wonderful remedy ; stew
red onions in fresh butter for an ointment : or beat the
juice of Stramonium or Jamestown leaves and wash
the part ; or burn English rosin in a pot, and get over it,
and take a small pill of opium on going to bed ; or drink
tar water, or take a cat and cut her throat and save
the blood, and skin her, then roast her, and save the
fat, then stew the blood and grease and a litle fine brim
stone, and apply this to the Piles, it is of great val
ue.

THE BILIOUS FEVER.

I will give a few general symptoms of this disease
it generally begins with a cold chill, pains in the limb
and back, and back of the neck and head, loss of appe
tite, then a high fever. In the beginning of any fever
the stomach is uneasy, vomit if the bowels purge ; i
the pulse be high or hard, full or strong, bleed and
drink thin water gruel sweetened with honey, with
one or two drachms of nitre to each quart. The best
drink in general, is to toast a large thin slice of bread
without burning, put it hot in cold water then set it on
coals and heat it well ; if the skin is dry, get a handful of white plantain, the same of cerqufoil, the same of
maidens hair, the same of polly pody, the same of
mountain tea, mix these all together and boil them,
use the tea for a constant drink, this will raise a mois-

ture upon the skin. Take pulverized brimstone twenty grains, ten grains of refined nitre, mix this together ; take five grains every four or five hours, until the fever subsides. If the pain in the head be violent, a blister should be drawn on the back of the neck. Should there be any pain in the breast, it will be necessary that a blister should be drawn on the pit of the stomach, and also on the inside of the legs above the ancles ; these blisters should be kept running by applying cabbage leaves. Get a handful of dogwood bark, the same of wild comfrey root, the same of catnip, boil these in a gallon of water to a pint, add to this, half a pint of madeira wine, ten grains of quinine or peruvian bark, the patient should take half a table spoonful three times per day. A solution of the cream of tartar and water should be the constant drink of the patient. If the patient should be in a costive habbit, Rhubarb, aloes, and calomel, should be freely given. I have given you a short account of the nature and treatment of this disease ; yet by attending to the same will be found of great advantage. .

THE CROUP.

This disease makes two important distinctions : the first is attended with spasm, and a dry cough ; the second is without spasm, and the patient under its influence, is able to cough up a considerable quantity of phlegm. The spasmodic croup comes on suddenly, and that generally in the night — has frequent and perfect intermissions of the symptoms for hours, and sometimes even for days, is attended with a dry cough as above, and is at last particularly relieved by the warm bath, asafœdita, opium, &c. To be more particular, the child will probably go to bed in perfect health, and in an our or two wake in a fright, with his face much flush-

ed or even of purple color, he will be unable to describe what he feels; will breath with much labor, and
a peculiar convulsive motion of the belly: his breathing will also be very quick, attended with a sound as if
he were threatened with a speedy suffocation. The
terror of the child increases his disorder, and he will
cling to the nurse, and if not speedily relieved by
coughing, sneezing, vomiting or purging, the suffocation will increase, the child will die. It is remarkable
that the cough in this disease very much resembles in
sound the barking of a young dog. There are also during the continuance of the disorder, frequent eruptions
of little red blotches on the skin, which for the time,
seem to afford relief; and this eruption will sometimes
appear and disappear two or three times, in the course
of the complaint. For the cure, in the first distinction
of the croup, the remedy is bleeding, when the difficnl-
ty is great, the face much flushed, or when the patient
expresses much pain in coughing, this remedy is absolutely necessary and should be repeated as often as
may be requisite. For subduing these symptoms, vomits, from five to ten grains of ipecacuanha, with two
or three grains of calomel may be given to a child from
two to four years old; or half a grain of tartar emetic,
with three or four grains of ipecacuanha; or five grains
of ipecacuanha with two or three grains of rhubarb, or
a tea spoonful of antimonial wine, or a spoonful of a
strong decoction of seneca, called also rattle snake
root; every dose used. it should be repeated till the
intended effect is produced. But bleeding ought first
to be performed. Jalap and calomel, from five to ten
grains of the former, with two or four of the latter,
may be given to a child of three to five, or six grains
or jalap eight to twelve grains, or castor oil; but this
is scarcely active enough for so violent a disease, the
warm bath may be used either before or after the bleeding; but it will be most effectual after the evacuations
and ought to be repeated daily for some time. Glys-

ers: milk and water, or chicken broth, or thin gruel may be used for this purpose; and in some instances, where the spasms remain after bleeding, &c. fifteen drops of the tincture of opium may be occasionally added to the injection; ten or fifteen grains of tartar emetic dissolved in half a pint of thin gruel or chicken broth — water is an excellent injection. Blisters will be found very serviceable after the evacuations of bleeding and purging; these may be applied to the back part of the neck, or to the side of the patient; when blisters are properly admissible, opium, asafœdita, &c., may be used with safety. The second distinction of this disorder is attended with symptoms very similar to those of the first; but may be known by its coming on gradually, and that commonly in the day time; by its continuing and frequently increasing for several days without any remarkable remission, or even abatement of the symptoms, by the discharge of phlegm. From the windpipe by coughing; as also by the appearance of slime in the stools, and lastly by its refusing to yield to the warm bath, opium, &c.

The remedies proper in this kind of croup are as before, but with some variations, bleeding when the breathing is difficult, the face flushed, the pulse light, &c., vomits, as under the first distinction, purges; but in these cases only calomel should be used. The principal dependence should be placed upon this medicine, a large dose should be given as soon as the disorder discovers itself. Six or eight grains to a child four years old, afterwards smaller doses should be given every day, so long as any of the symptoms continue, from two to four grains might answer this intention. It is important that relief should be afforded; the first attack of this violent disease, if neglected, it will be fatal in almost every instance, &c. I often have found benefit from this medicine: that is get an egg, or take the white and a piece of alum as big as a Partridge egg, and beat it fine take the same quantity of beat brimstone, mix them together and take the clear water that comes from that, and give them a little now and then; this will dry them out immediately, or scarify them between the shoulders and catch the blood and mix with breast milk, and give them to drink; this has relieved many of the hives, &c.

PROLAPSUS UTERI.

This complaint consists (as the name implies) in a change of the situation of the womb, by which this organ falls much lower than it ought to do. In some cases, it absolutely protrudes entirely without the vagina. The slighter cases are therefore named a bearing down, and the more violent ones a descent, or falling down of the Uterus. The complaint is met with in women of every age: but more frequently in those who have had several children, than in such as have not had any. Every disease which induces general debility, or local weakness in the passage leading to the womb in particular may lay the foundation of this complaint; hence, frequent miscarriages, improper treatment during labor, too early or violent exercise after delivery, immoderate venery, &c., are, in married women, the most frequent circumstances by which a bearing or falling down of the womb is produced. In the unmarried, it is apt to take place in consequence of violent exertions, such as jumping, dancing, riding, lifting heavy weights, &c., while out of order. The disease comes on generally with an uneasy sensation in the loins whilst standing or walking, accompanied now and then with a kind of pressure and bearing down. By disregarding these feelings, the woman becomes at length incapable of making water without first lying down or pushing up the swelling which seems to impede the discharge of urine, and if the complaint continues to increase, the womb is actually forced out of the parts, and takes on the form of a bulky substance hanging down between the thighs. This severe degree of the disorder seldom occurs, however, among women in northern climates, except in those who have had many children, and are at the same time of a relaxed and feeble frame; but in warm climates it is frequently to be met with, and particularly in negroes and mulatoes, among whom I often observed the protruded parts considerably ulcerated, and occasioned no doubt by neglect of cleanliness, and external irritation. Although prolapsus uteri is a local disease, it is frequently productive of several distressing symptoms which undermine the constitution. These principally arise from disturbed functions of the stomach and bowels, and an impaired condition of the nervous system.— When of long standing, it will be difficult to effect a cure. In the treatment of this complaint, the means must be adapted to the degree of its violence. When the case is of a recent nature, and the descent inconsiderable, an invigorating diet with horse exercise, the daily use of a cold bath, both general and local, and the injection of some mild astringent such as, a solution of borax, gum kino, red oak bark, &c. If there is great difficulty of making water, a strong tea of parsley or horsemint should be daily used, the back and hips should be bathed frequently in buzzards oil, if the bowels are costive, the cream of tartar, jalap, or Rhubarb, should be frequently used. Should there be any fever, a strong decoction of slippery elm bark should be daily used, the tincture of cubebs should be used from ten to thirty drops a day in a little water. Should the abdomen or belly become swelled, a weak solution of the sugar of lead may be cautiously used. By pursuing this course of treatment there is no difficulty of the patient deing relieved, &c.

EPISTAXIS, OR HEMORRHAGE FROM THE NOSE.

In the nose there is a considerable net-work of blood vessels expanded on the internal surface of the nostrils, and covered only with a thin tegument; hence, upon any determination of a greater quantity of blood than is ordinary to the vessels of the head, those of the nose are easily ruptured. In general, the blood flows only from one nostril; but in some cases it is discharged from both, then showing a more considerable disease. Persons of a sanguine and plethoric habit, and not yet advanced to manhood, are very liable to be attacked with the complaint; females being much less subject to it than males, particularly after menstruation has commenced. Peculiar weaknes in the vessels of the part, and the decline of life, may also be considered as predisposing causes. Great heat, violent exertion, external violence, particular postures of the body, and, every thing that determines the blood to the head, are to be looked upon as its exciting cause.

Epistaxis, comes on at times, without any previous warning; but at others, it is preceded by a pain and heaviness in the head, vertigo, tinnitus, aurium, flushing in the face, heat and itching in the nostrils, a throbbing of the temporal arteries, and a quickness of the pulse. In some instances, a coldness of the feet, and shivering over the whole body, together with a costive belly, are observed to precede an attack of the hemorrhage. The complaint is to be considered as of little consequence when occurring in young persons, being seldom attended with danger; but when it aiises in those more advanced in life, flows profusely, and returns frequently, it indicates too great a fullness of the vessels in the head and not unfrequently precedes apoplexy, palsy, &c., and therefore such cases are to be regarded as a dangerous disease. When this hemorrhage arises in any putrid disorder, it is to be considered as a fatal symptom. As a bleeding from the nose proves salutary in some disorders, such as vertigo, and head-ache, and is critical in others such as phrenzy, apoplexy and inflammatory, where there is a determination of too great a quantity of blood to the head, we ought properly to consider at the time it happens, whether it is really a disease, or intended by nature to remove some other—when it arises in the course of some inflammatory disorder, or in any other where we have reasons to suspect too great determination of blood to the head, we should suffer it to go on so long as the patient is not weakened by it, neither should it be suddenly stopped when it happens to persons in good health who are of a full and plethoric habit. When it arises in elderly people or returns too frequently or continues till the patient becomes faint, it ought to be stopped immediately. To effect this, the person is to be exposed freely to cool air, the head should be bathed in cold water, a snuff should be immediately prepared, that is, take one ounce of bucks horn burned and finely pulverized, half an ounce of Indian turnip prepared in the same way, five grains of refined nitre pulverized fine, this should be well mixed together and used as snuff frequently. A little ether should also be frequently poured on the head, a little common table salt, and tobacco snuff, this may also at times be used when the case is very violent, a blister may be drawn on the back of the neck, the temples may also be cupped. The patient should also drink freely of cooling liquors. Where it arises in young people, the head should be held over the smoke of chicken feathers, and the same course pursued as above mentioned. A snuff prepared of cranes-bill or alum root, and used as the other preparation, is good in hemorrhage of the nose, and no doubt will give relief. As I have mentioned different kinds of hemorrhage it will not be necessary to make any further remarks at this time.

HEMORRHAGE, OR INVOLUNTARY DISCHARGE OF BLOOD.

Under this title are comprehended active hemorrhages, only, that is, those attended with some degree o
symptoms of the blood in the vessels from which it flows,
chiefly arising from an internal cause. On venesection
the blood appears as in the case of phlegmasiae ; that
is, the gluten sepeiated, or a crust formed. The general iemote causes of hemorrhages of this nature, are,
external heat, a sanguine and plethoric habit, whatever
increases the force of the circulation, as violent exercise, strong exertions, anger, and other active passions,
particular postures of the body, ligatures producing local congestion, a determination to certain vessels, rendered habitual from the frequent repetion of hemorrhage, the suppression of accustomed evacuations, external violence, and exposure to cold. The general
treatment of such hemorrhages must consist in putting
a stop to the discharge of the blood, in preventing its
recurrence, by iemoving the causes by which they
were excited, and by destroying the inflammatory diathesis when any exist. These means remain to be
pointed out under each distinct hemorrhage, as in the
subsequent pages.

SYNOCHA, OR INFLAMMATORY FEVER.

Syncha is a fever with much increased heat; a frequent, strong and hard pulse ; the urine red ; the animal functions but little disturbed, although at an advanced stage the sensoiium is apt to become much affected, it makes its attack at all seasons of the year, but
is most prevalent in the spring ; and it seizes persons
of all ages and habits, but more particularly those in
the vigor of life, with strong eleastic fibres, and a plethoric constitution. It is a species of fever almost pecu-

liar to cold and temperate climates, being rarely met
with in very warm ones, except among Europeans late-
ly arrived ; and even then the inflammatory stage is of
short duration, as it soon assumes the typhoid type.

The exciting causes are, sudden transitions from heat
to cold, the application of cold to the body when warm,
swallowing cold liquors when much heated by exercise, too free a use of vinous and spirituous liquors, great
intemperance, violent passions of the mind, exposure to
the rays of the sun, tropical inflammation, the suppression of habitual evacuations, the drying up of old
ulcers, and the sudden repulsion of eruptions. It may
be doubted if this fever ever originates from personal
infection ; but it is possible for it to appear pretty
generally among such as are of a robust habit, from a
peculiar state of the atmosphere. It comes on with a
sense of lassitude and inactivity, succeeded by vertigo,
rigors and pains over the whole body, but more particularly in the head and back ; which symptoms are
shortly followed by redness of the face, throbbing of
the temples, great restlessness, intence heat, and un-
quenchable thirst, oppression of breathing, and nausea. The skin is dry and parched ; the eyes appear
nflamed, and are incapable of bearing the light, the
tongue is of a scarlet color at the sides, and furred
with white in the centre ; the urine is red and scanty
the body is costive, and there is a quickness,. with a
fullness and hardness in the pulse, not much affected
by any pressure made on the artery. Its pulsations are
from ninety to one hundred and thirty ir a min and
when blood is taken, it exhibits a yellowish lymph or
buffy crust on its surface, which is the coagulable
lymph of febrine. If the febrile symptoms run very
high, and proper means are not used at an early period,
stupor and delirium comes on at a more dvanced
stage, the imagination becomes much distuabed and
hurried, and the patient raves violently. The disease
usually goes through its course in about fourteen days,

and terminates critically, either by a diaphoresis, diarrhœa, hemorrhage from the nose, or the deposits of a
copious sediment in the urine ; which crisis is generally preceeded by some variation in the pulse. In
some instances, it, however, terminates fatally. Our
judgement as to the termination of the disease must be
formed from the violence of the attack, and the nature
of the symptoms. If the fever runs high, or continues
many days, with great action of the heart and arteries, flushed turgid face, and red eyes, intolerance of
light, with vertigo or early stupor and delirium, the
event may be doubtful ; but if to these are added,
picking at the bed clothes, starting of the tendons, in-
volutary discharges by stool and urine and hickups, it
will then certainly be fatal. On the contrary, if the febrile heat abates, and the other symptoms moderate,
and there is a tendency to a crisis, which is marked
by an universal and natural perspiration on the body ;
by the urine depositing a lateritious sediment, and by
the pulse becoming more slow or soft ; or by a hemorrhage from the nose ; diarrhœa supervening ; or the
formation of abscesses ; we may then expect a recovery.
In a few cases, this fever has been succeded by mania,
in many instances, as there appear to be a general debility of the system, and a considerable inflammation.
It will be very necessary that the inflammation be allayed as soon as possible, it is very frequently the case,
that the inflammation appears to be confined to a particular part of the system, at times in the head, sometimes in the breast, when it is confined to the head, the
feet and hands are generally cold, the general circulation of the blood when this is the case is generally confined to the part that is most affected, instead of flowing to the extremities, the first thing necessary in this
case is to endeavor to produce a regular flow of blood
through the system, and endeavor as much as possible
to keep down the inflammation. Ten grains of ipecacuanha combined with one drop of the oil of croton,

this should be given in a little warm water. If it does not produce vomiting in the course of thirty minutes, five grains more of the ipecacuanha should be given, it should be worked off with warm water and gruel, so soon as it is done operating, purgatives such as rhubarb, mandrake, senna, should be freely used, if the fever should be high bleeding is necessary, if. pain should be great, blistering will also be necessary, on the back of the neck, on the ancles and the inside of the legs—If the case should be very violent and no relief found from the above remedies. Five grains of calomel, combined with three grains of jalap, one of gambouge, this should be given every night, or oftener if necessary, until it produces an expectoration from the Saliva glands, mild tonics should also be used, such as barks quinine, &c.

CHILDREN, OR LOOSENESS OF THE BOWELS.

Various causes may and do occasion a diarrhœa in infants, and perhaps in the greater number of instances, it is brought on, either by too much or unsuitable food, in which cases a diligent attention must be paid both to the choice and regulation of the diet. In some instances however, it may be symptomatic of other diseases, or however, it may arise from an exposure to cold, or an increased secretion of bile. In the latter case, it may be advisable first of all to cleanse the stomach by a gentle emetic, but in all, it will be proper to clear the intestines by a few grains of rhubarb and magnesia, the operation of which being over we, may give a little of the prepared chalk, joined with some aromatic, twice or thrice a day. When the stools continue to be more frequent than they ought to be, and are either slimy or tinged with blood, it will be necessary to repeat the rhubarb at proper intervals, and in the mean time the infant may take something to con-

trol the complaint, as well as proper nutriment to re-
cruit its strength. Flour, sage, or rice boiled in milk,
together with the jelly of a calf's foot or isinglass,
with a small addition of wine, will be good articles of
diet under such circumstances. In addition to these
means it will be advisable to envelope the infants body
in flannel, so as to keep it of a proper temperature.
That form of diarrhœa which is attended by green
stools and griping, may in general be removed readily
by a brisk laxative, consisting of the submuriate of
mercury, and rhubarb, followed by small doses of magnesia and chalk. When obstinate, we may give half a
grain of calomel, or three grains of rhubarb or jalap,
or mandrake, the applications of a blister to the pit of
the stomach may be necessary. A few drops of the
tincture of opium may be given, also the oil of peppermint in small quantities may be given. The external
application of opium and the sugar of lead is also good.

GUTTA SERENA AMAUROSIS OR DIMNESS OF SIGHT.

Gutta serena, (a species of blindness wherein the
eyes remain fair and seemingly unaffected,) consists
in a dimness of sight, whether the object be near or at
a distance, together with the representation of flies,
dust, &c., floating before the eyes; and the pupil is
generally deprived of its power of contraction. It is
supposed to depend on some of the optic nerves; but
its causes are, nevertheless, said to be various.; some
of which are, from their nature, incapable of being removed. Thus, in one case, the blindness has been
found to be occasioned by an encysted tumor, which
was situated in the substance of the cerebrum, and
pressed on the optic nerves near their origin: in a second, by a cist, containing a considerable quantity of
water, and lodging itself on the optic nerves, at the

part where they unite : in a third, by a caries of the
os-frontis, occasioning an alteration in the optic for a
midd ; and in a fourth, by malformation of the optic
nerves themselves.   In some cases the defect of vision
has been attempted to be accounted for, by supposing
a defect in the optic nerves, disqualifying them for
conveying the impression of objects through the eyes
to the brain, as, upon the minutest inspection by dissection, nothing has been discovered, either in the
structure of the eyes, or in the state of any of the
component parts contributing to the faculty of vision,
which could at all obstruct the performance of their
proper office.   Mr. Ware, in his treaties on this disease, mentions that a dilation of the arterial circle, surrounding the cella turciea, (which is formed by the ca-
rotid arteries on each side, by branches passing from
them to meet each other before, and by other branches
passing backward to meet branches from the basilary
artery behind,) may likewise be a cause of gutta serena.   The anterior portion of this circle passes over
the optic nerves. which, undoubtedly, may therefore
become compressed when any enlargement of these
vessels takes place.

Having made a few general remarks on the nature
and symptoms of this disease, we will now pursue a
general course of treatment which I consider to be
beneficial in the cure of the same.   Its treatment is
usually regulated on the plan of stimulating either the
parts themselves or the system in general.   The first
that should be done is to apply blisters or issues to the
back of the neck, at the same time a solution of pulverised ginger and senna should be used frequently, so
as to keep the bowels entirely free and open.   It is
very necessary that blood should be taken from the
arm every third or fourth day, in small quantities ; epsom salts should be frequently used.   The head should
also be bathed in a solution of sulphuratic either, sugar
of lead and water ; the bead should be bathed in it all

over, once every day; the diet should be of the most limited kind, and a dark room should confine the patient. No exposure whatever to the damp or wet air: by pursuing this general course of treatment, the patient may be relieved of this sad and unfortunate disease.

CHRONIC RHEUMATISM.

This disease may arise at any time of the year. The characteristics of rheumatism, as assigned by Dr. Cullen, are pains in the muscles, joints, knees, ancles, &c. When there are frequent vicissitudes of the weather, from hot to cold, it generally gives rise to this disease. But the spring and autumn are the seasons in which it is most prevalent, and it attacks persons of all ages, but very young people are more exempt from it than adults. Those whose employments subject them to alterations of heat and cold, are particularly liable to rheumatism. Although acute rheumatism somewhat resembles the gout, still, in some respects, it differs from it. It does not usually come on so suddenly as a fit of the gout, but for the most part gives the patient warning by a slow and gradual increase of pain. Neither is it fixed to one spot like the gout, but is distinguished by its frequent wanderings from place to place, accompanied by a sense of numbness. It seldom attacks the small joints, but is confined chiefly to the larger, as the hip, knees and shoulders. Acute rheumatism is generally attended with a continued fever; whereas the gout has periodical remissions. Like most of pyrexiae, it is preceded by rigors and sense of cold. A febrile, quick and hard pulse supervenes: the veins near the part affected swell, and a throbbing pain is felt in the arteries. By degrees the pain increases, and the patient suffers cruel torture, which is increased on the least motion. The sense of pain resembles that of a slow dilaceration of the parts, and commonly goes off by a swelling of the joint or joints. The rheumatism moreover is not preceded by dyspeptic symptoms, as is usually the case with the gout; neither do chalky concretions form about the small joints and fingers as in the latter.

Obstructed perspiration, occasioned either by wearing wet clothes, lying in damp linen, sleeping on the ground or in damp rooms, or by being exposed to cool air when the body has been much heated by exercise or by coming from a crowded public place into the cool air, is the cause which usually produces rheumatism. Those who are much afflicted with this complaint are very apt to be sensible of the approach of wet weather, by finding wandering pains about them at that period: More particularly the chronic, is attended with pains in the head, shoulders, knees, and other large joints, which at times are confined to one particular part, and at others shift from one joint to another without occasioning any inflammation or fever, and in this manner the complaint continues often for a considerable time, and at length goes off, leaving the parts which have been affected in a state of debility, and very liable to fresh impressions on the approach of moist damp weather. Little danger is attended on chronic rheumantism; but a person having been attacked with it, is ever afterwards more or less liable to returns of it, there being some of the general symptoms laid before the reader, he can discover the difference between chronic and acute rheumatism, as the acute is generally confined to one joint in particular, as there is such a difference between acute and chronic, there is no difficulty in deciding the case. As the system is generally debilitated from chronic inflammation, it is necessary that the digestive powers of the stomach, with a general perspiration of the system should be attended to, this should be done by the following preparation — ten grains of calomel, two of tartarized antimony, three grains of cayenne pepper, one grain of gum camphor, this should be dissolved in a little ginger tea, this should be taken at night and worked off with a little chicken soup or gruel — when the pain is great blisters should be drawn on the back of the neck, ancles and wrists, when there is any fever, bleeding is necessary; a strong tea, of Lignumvitæ should be frequently given. The joints should be rubbed with the spirits of turpentine and camphor combined together. If the bowels are costive the daily use of the tincture of rhubarb or Peruvian bark should be resorted to as a promoter of the same. The patient should take from a half to a table spoonful of the tincture of gum guiaccum, three times a day, in a little water, if the pain in the breast be considerable a small pill of opium may at times be taken, avoiding cold or night air, the diet should be limited. By pursuing this course you may be relieved of this distressing complaint. In case of the acute, the joints should be well steamed with a still cap, and alcohol, and the above treatment should be strictly attended to in the mean while.

N. B. The alcohol should be set under the cap of the still and set on fire — and the arm of the cap placed so as to conduct the steam to the affected part, the patient should be covered with a blanket, and drink strong teas while going through this operation.

ABORTIONS.

By abortion is to be understood the expulsion of the contents of the gravid uterus at a period of gestation, so early as to render it impossible for the fœtus to live. It is an accident or disease of frequent occurrence, which is always attended with disagreeable circumstances, and which, although it seldom proves immediately fatal, may still be productive of much mischief at a future period. Abortions may happen at any period of

pregnancy, but they take place more frequently about
the third or fourth month. From the end of the third
month to the period of quickening, there is a greater
susceptibility in the uterus to have its action interrupted than either before or afterwards, which is the reason of more miscarriages happening at that time than
at any other, and points out the necessity of re-
doubling our vigilence in watching and guarding against
the operations of any of the causes from the tenth to
the sixteenth week, that may be likely to excite abortion. When a woman happens to part with her bur-
den before the seventh month, she is said to have
miscarried or aborted; but when delivered of it after
this time, the term labor is usually applied. Children
born at the end of the seventh month are seldom reared,
and when they are, they usually prove small and weakly; but those of eight months are frequently preserved
by bestowing proper care on them. In consequence
of an imperfect conception, it sometimes happens that
moles or substances of a fleshy nature (which upon being cut open contain not the smallest vestige of a child)
are formed in the uterus; and these at length becoming detached, give rise to a considerable degree of hemorrhage. As some women menstruate during the
first months of pregnancy, it will be necessary to distinguish between an approaching miscarriage and a
visitation of the menses, which may readily be done by
inquiring whether or not the hemorrhage has proceeded from any evident case, and whether it flows gently
or is accompanied with unusual pains.

The former generally arises from some fright, surprise, or accident, and does not flow gently and regularly, but bursts out of a sudden, and again stops all at
once, and is also attended with severe pains in the back
and bottom of the belly; whereas the latter is marked
with no such occurrences. Voluptuous women who
are of a weak and irritable frame, are most apt to miscarry; but accidents of this nature sometimes occur

from a general defective constitution, or from a mal-
conformation of the sexual organs. The causes which
give rise to floodings during a state of pregnancy, are
violent exertions of strength, lifting some heavy weight,
severe exercise, as dancing or much walking, the fa-
tiguing dissipations of fashionable life, sudden surpri-
ses, frights, violent fits of passion, great uneasiness of
mind, uncommon longing, over-fulness of blood, partial
spasmodic action about the os-uteri, alœtic purges, profuse evacuations, excessive venery, former miscarriages,
weakness in the parts immediately concerned, a diseased state of the uterus, general debility of the system, external injuries, as blows and bruises, strong and
acrid medicines, such as savin and hellebore, which are
often taken for the express purpose of exciting abortion, and the death of the child. A pregnant woman
may be attacked with a flow of blood from the womb
in consequence of any cause which is capable of sepa-
rating a part of the ovum from the corresponding part
of the uterus. The vessels which before passed straight
from its internal surface into the membranes or placenta, and connected them together, now open, so as
to allow the blood to escape between them, and to flow
externally. This separation and consequent rupture
may arise from any of the causes just recited, but in a
few instances, it is occasioned by an implantation of a
part of the placenta immediately over the os-uteri,
which cause is by far the most important, because it is
most dangerous, and the least likely to find a spontaneous remedy. Abortions are sometimes induced by
what is termed a retroversion of the uterus, in which
the fundus uteri is retroverted and passed down between
the rectum and vagina, this rarely occurs, however, beyond the first or second month of gestation, and is generally preceded by a difficulty in making water, and a
consequent tumor of the bladder; a violent pain about
the perinæum is thus caused, and a miscarriage is likely
to follow.

Abortions are often preceded by a general sense of coldnes; flacidity of the breasts, slight pains in the loins, and lower region of the belly ; and sometimes with a slight febrile state of the system. In plethoric habits and where abortion proceeds from over-action or hemorrhagic action of the uterine vessels, the fever is idiopathic, and preceeds the hemorahage. After a short continuance of these symptoms, a slight discharge of blood ensues, coming away sometimes in clots, and at others, gushing out in a florid stream, then stopping perhaps for a short time, and again returning violently. On the first appearance of a flooding, the woman should be confied to her bed, and be placed with her hips somewhat more elevated than her head, keeping her at the sametime cool, debaring her of all food of a heating or stimulent nature, and giving her cold liquors to drink sharpened with some agreegable acid.   With a view of moderating the symptoms attending the progress of a threatened abortion, and preventing it if possible, from actually taking place, it may be proper in robust and plethoric habits, and where the pulse is in any degree full and frequent, to take away a little blood from the arm, after which, if the bowels are confined, we may administer a laxative clyster. If the discharges ar copious the bowels should be kept bathed in strong vinegar; at the same time, five grains of the following powders should be taken every twenty minutes ; take of kino one ounce, alum the same and the same of cinnamon, bark, also one ounce of the inside bark of black gum, the same of angelica seed, the same of the inside bark of dogwood, let these be well pulverised together to a fine powder. and taken as directed in a little water, this course should be pursued until the violence of the case is somewhat abated.   It should then be taken in less quantities and not so often ; a few drops of laudanum may at times be given ; the bowels in the meantime kept moderately open, by mild purgatives such as the following take of salts one ounce, manna half an ounce, tincture of rhubarb one ounce, let these be mixed together, the patient should take half a table spoonful as often as the case may require in cold spring water. If the bowels appear to be swelled from any inflammation, one grain of the sugar of lead may be administered once or twice a day. The bowels should also be well bathed once or twice a day in a solution of sulphuric ether and water. If the courses should be stopped too suddenly, a little stimulous should be used, but should be done very cautiously, a little wine or weak tody may in all probability have the desired effect, if given several times as needful.

HEMOPTYSIS, OR SPITTING OF BLOOD.

In hemoptyses there is a discharge of blood of a florid color, and often frothy, from the mouth, brought up with more or less coughing or hawking, and preceded usually by a saltish taste in the saliva, a sense of weight about the precordia, difficult respiration and a pain in some part of the thorax. It is readily to be distinguished from the hematemesis, as in this last, the blood is usually thrown up in considerable quantities, is moreover of a dark color, more gumous, and mixed with the other contents of the stomach, and is unattended by any cough; whereas blood proceeding from the lungs is usually in small quantity, is of a florid color, fluid mixed with a little frothy mucus, and brought up by coughing. A spitting of blood arises most usually between the age of sixteen and twenty-five, and may be occasioned by any violent exertion, either in running jumping, wrestling, singing, speaking loud, or blowing wind instruments; as likewise by wounds, plethora, pneumonia, weak vessels, hectic fever, coughs irregular living, excessive drinking, or the suppression of some accustomed discharge, such as the menstrual or hemorrhoidal. It may be occasioned by breathing air which is too much rarified, to be able properly to

expand the lungs. Persons in whom there is a faulty
proportion either of the vessels of the lungs, or in the
capacity of the chest, being distinguished by a narrow
thorax and prominent shoulders, or who are of a delicate make and sanguine temperament, or who have had
previous affections of the same disease, seem much
predisposed to this hemorrhage ; but in these the complaint is often brought on by the concurrence of various occasional and exciting causes before mentioned.
A spitting of blood is not, however, always to be considered as a primary disease. It is often only a symptom, and in some disorders, such as pleuresies, pcrip-
neumonies, and many fevers, often arises, and is the pre-
sage of a favorable termination, if only very slight.
Sometimes it is preceded (as has already been observed) by a sense of weight and oppression at the chest,
a dry tickling cough, some slight difficulty of breathing and a hard jerking pulse. At other times it is ush-
ered in with shiverings, coldness of the extremities,
pains in the back and loins, fletulency, costiveness, and
lassitude. The blood which is spit up is sometimes thin,
and of a florid red color; and at other times it is thick,
and of a dark or blackish cast; nothing, however. can
be inferred from this circumstance, but that the blood
has lain a longer or shorter time in the chest before it
was discharged.

It seldom takes place to such a degree as to prove
fatal at once, but when it does, the effusion is from some
large vessel. The danger, therefore, will be in proportion as the discharge of blood comes from a large vessel or small one, and as the quantity is profuse or trifling. When the disease proves fatal in consequence of
the rupture of some large vessel, there is found on dissection a considerable quantity of clotted blood between the lungs and pleura, and there is usually more
or less of an inflammatory appearance at the ruptured
part. Where the disease terminates in pulmonary
consumption, the same morbid appearances are to be

met with as described under that particular head, &c. As the general symptoms of this complaint are laid before the reader, we shall in the next place proceed to the treatment of the same. The first thing necessary is to produce that regular action of the lungs that nature requires. this may be done by astringent medicines such as the following:— Take half an ounce of pulverised cinnamon bark the same of gum kino, the same of cubebs, add these articles together, in one pint of alcohol, let it stand for three days, the patient should take of this a half a tea spoonful three times a day combined with honey, this course of treatment should be pursued for several days. The patient should also take a tea spoonful of sweet oil every morning combined with two grains of loaf sugar and five drops of laudanum, the constant drink should be a weak solution of the cream of tartar combined with a small portion of the sugar of lead, if the bowels are costive the patient should use the tincture of aloes, or a strong tea of peach tree leaves, should there be any fever bleeding will be also necessary. If the stomach appear weak and much debilitated, a few drops of elixir vitriol should be used in a little weak tody two or three times a day. A small pill of opium may at times be taken. The head should be frequently bathed in cold water. The diet should be limited, &c. I have laid down a few prescriptions and if the patient attends to them strictly he may be relieved.

ODONTALIGIA, OR TOOTH ACHE.

The tooth-ache consists in an acute pain in one or more of the teeth; but most generally it originates in one, and from that is diffused to the adjacent parts. A caries of the tooth itself, acted upon by different irritating causes, such as the application of cold, or some ac-

8

rid matter, are the most usual causes of this complaint;
but in some cases it would seem to proceed from a rheu-
matic affection of the muscles and membranes of the
jaw; and here the whole side of the face will he affected.   When it takes place in pregnanc y, it is to be
considered as arising either from an increased irritability or from sympathy.   It may be presumed that the
acrid matter which occasions the tooth-ache, is produced
by some vice that originates in the tooth itself.   In
some instances the caries appears first upon the external surface or enamel of the tooth, in one or more
spots which are superficial; but in others it commences
in the internal surface or long part: The former is,
however, by far the most frequent.   The caries, by spreading and corroding deeper, at length penetrates the substance of the tooth; and the external air, and other matters getting into the cavity; stimulate the nerve, & thereby excite the tooth-ache. The most effectual cure for this
disease is extraction of the carious tooth; but as this in
some cases may not be advisable, and in others might
be strongly objected to by the patient, it will often be
necessary to substitute paliative means.   The oil of
pepper, combined with the tincture of opium should
frequently be used, that is, put it on a piece of cotton
and put the same frequently in the hollow of the tooth.
The oil of peneroyal combined with the oil of cloves may
be used in the same way. If the above preparations sho'd
fail giving relief, a few drops of nitric-acid may be applied in the same manner as the above.   If there be no
hollow in the tooth, there may be a few drops of laudanum, or alcohol, French brandy or sweet oil—either
of these droped in the ear, on the side affected will relieve the pain immediately.

> I am sure this will cure,
> If properly applied;
> It's not hard, for to indure,
> It's been frequently tried.

FOR A MORTIFICATION.

Apply a poultice of flour, honey and water, with a little yeast. When a mortification takes place, the flesh is not already dead, but is dying, or in a state of dying. It is often necessary to abate it by bleeding, if the fever admits, and by cooling, opening medicines: The parts around touched with vinegar, lime water, or camphorated spirits, and scarrified ; apply a poultice of biscuit of fine wheat flour, boiled with miik to the mortified place, and take the bark freely ; or apply puccoon juice and honey—this is wonderful ; or make a poultice of dogwood bark, black oak bark, sassafras bark, black haw bark, sumac roots, and wheat flour or rye meal, and bathe the place before hand, with bitter herbs ; or take some tar, feathers, brimstone and hickory coals and put in a vessel and hold the mortified place over the steam—this is wonderful.

THE CRAMP COLIC.

This is a colic that cramps the stomach, and draws the patient sometimes nearly double with violent pains all through the breast, and will roll through the bowel' like goose eggs, and sometimes goes off with a lax, o discharge of wind, up or down, before the patient can get any ease. Parched peas, eaten freely, have had a happy effect, when other means have failed ; a gill of dogwood berries, boiled in a quart of water down to half a pint, and drank, is wonderful ; or boil a large burdoc leaf in a quart of water to a gill, and drink ; or take and scrape the inside of a pipe: soot water, or weak lye is very good ; or take a teaspoonful of pulverized charcoal in a little water and drink this ; or take a young shoat and cut it open in haste, and obtain the gall and drink — it may probably relieve the patient ; or make ginger tea and drink ; or take cala-

mus, chew and swallow the spittle ; or eat ginger root
freely ; or combine a small quantity of aloes, asafœdita
and rhubarb, put these in spirits and drink as needful.
But of all medicines I have ever used, is garlic boiled
in new milk, this prescription often relieves the quickest
of any remedy that has ever been tried.   Beware of
eating such food as creates wind or is hard of digestion.

      This disease is very bad,
      And cramps the patient up,
      And if a cure cannot be had,
      You'll soon be drawn enough.

THE MENSES, &c.

There is a certain periodical evacuation which takes
place with all healthy females, beginning when they
arrive at twelve or fifteen years of age, and continuing
until forty-five or fifty.   This I cannot call a disease, as
it is universal to the sex ; and as there cannot be health
without it, you should begin in due time to instruct
your daughters in the conduct and management of
themselves.   At this critical time of life, a few lessons
seasonably given, may prevent much mischief.   But
little attention is necessary to know when this discharge
is about to commence.   There are particular symptoms
which go before it, and foretell its approach ; as a sense
of heat and weight, with a dull pain in the loins, a
swelling and hardness of the breast, head ache, loss of
appetite, uncommon weakness of the limbs, paleness of
the countenance, and sometimes a slight degree of fever.   Whenever these symptoms appear about the age
at which the terms begin to flow, every thing that obstructs it must be carefully avoided, and such means
used as tend to bring it forward.   She should sit over
the steam of warm water, bathing her feet at the same
time in a vessel filled with the same, and so deep as to
reach up to her knees.   She should drink freely of

warm, diluting liquors, such as weak flax seed tea, mallow or balm teas, or sweat over bitter herbs. The most proper time for these things is the evening, so that she may cover herself up warmly in bed after the bathing, and after continuing the drink until bed time, &c. Some precautions, however, are necessary, before the symptoms which usher in this discharge, present themselves. For if she be closely confined about this time, and be not engaged in some active employment, which may give proper exercise to her whole body, she will become weak, relaxed and sickly, her countenance will be pale, her spirits will sink, her vigor decline, and she, perhaps, will become weakly and sickly the remainder of her life. It is often the case that the daughters of the fashionable and wealthy, who, according to custom, have been much indulged, entirely give themselves up to indolence at this critical time, and bring upon themselves such irregularities as render them miserable for life. We seldom meet with complaints from cold, as it is commonly called, among active and industrious girls ; while, on the contrary, the ndolent and slothful are seldom free from them, A sprightly disposition, and a habitual cheerfulness ought to be cultivated with all possible attention, not only as conductive to prevent obstructions, but as the best defence against vapors and hysterics. The cheerfulness, however, which I here recommend, is not mere mirth and laughter, it is a calm and uniform serenity which prepares a rational being, thankfully and heartily to enjoy the real comforts of life ; it is a peculiar spring which gives to the mind as much activity when in retirement, as in a ball room. Towards this time, every thing which has a tendency to impair digestion and derange the regular motions of the system, ought to be avoided ; such as eating largely, or brash, light clothes, loss of sleep and excessive exercise, To this last, we may generally affix dancing, change of clothes without proper regard being had to their degree of warmth, is frequently productive of mischief; occasional exposure of the skin to cool air, if continued but a short time only, seldom does injury. But a great change in the clothes, from warm to cool, is frequently very pernicious; changes of this kind ought to be brought about in a gradual manner. I have known serious effects from too long exposure of the feet to wet and cold.

Country girls frequently·wade through the water, walk barefoot in the morning, and sit without door for hours in the evening, &c. Either of these acts may do irreparable damage, whether about the time of the first flowing of the menses, or at any time of its return. Indeed such exposure as at another time might produce no ill effects, may, at this juncture, be followed by irreparable damage to her health. But after all your care, it will sometimes happen that the courses will not begin to flow at that period of life when they usually make their appearance. Should this be the case, and in consequence of their retention her health and spirits begin to decline, by no means be persuaded to confine her to her room, nor expect to restore her by heat and medicine only. Instead of confinement, carry her abroad into agreeable company; turn her attention to some interesting employment; let her eat plentifully of wholesome food, and promote its digestion by taking regularly a sufficient portion of exercise; and in most instances nature will do her own work without any other assistance than that above. And after pursuing this plan a sufficient length of time without success, you will be at liberty to have recource to medicine, and the medicine well directed according to the complaint, as the symptoms stated in the directions of the difficulty of menstruation with pain, &c. Sometimes the retention is the consequence of an imperforated hymen; when this is the case, it may be felt with the finger, and should be pierced with a proper instrument; for this purpose a surgeon should be employed.

A SUPPRESSION OF THE MENSES.

Any interruption occurring after the menstrual flux has once been established in its regular course except when occasioned by conception, is always to be considered as a case of suppression. A constriction of the extremities of the vessels of the uterus, arising from accidental circumstances, such as cold, anxiety of mind, fear, inactivity of body, the frequent use of acids and other sedatives, &c., is the cause which evidently produces a suppression of the menses. In some few cases it appears as a symptom of other diseases, and particularly of general debility in the system. Herein there is a want of the necessary propelling force or due action of the vessels. When the menstrual flux has been suppressed for any considerable length of time, it not unfrequently happens that the blood which should have passed off by the uterus, being determined more copiously and perfectly to other parts, gives rise to hemorrhages: hence it is frequently poured out from the nose, stomach, lungs, and other parts in such cases. At first, however, febrile or inflammatory symptoms appear, the pulse is hard and frequent, the skin hot, and there is a severe pain in the head, back, and loins; besides being subject to these occurrences, the patient is likewise much troubled with costiveness, colic pains, and with dyspeptic and hysteric symptoms. Our prognostic in this disease is to be directed by the cause which has given rise to it, the length of time it has continued and the state of the persons health in other respects. When suddenly suppressed in consequence of cold it may easily be removed by pursuing proper means; but where the suppression has been of long standing, and lucorrhœa attends, we ought always to consider such circumstances as unfavorable. In those cases which have terminated fatally, in consequence of the long continuance of the disease, the same morbid changes in the ovaria and uterus are to be observed on dissection, as in those of a retention of the menses. What we are principally to have in view in the treatment of this complaint, is to remove (if possible) the constriction which effect the extremities of the vessels of the uterus; and this is to be done with the use of relaxants, where these or most of these symptoms occur, take blood from the foot ten or twelve ounces, to be repeated as occasion may require, the feet should be bathed in warm water, a portion of calomel and aloes may also be given — abstain from heavy draughts of cold water, the calomel and aloes may be given every third night, and live on light diet and keep from cold. Bleeding is very necessary in this case, and if there should be any swelling of the feet and ancles or a bloating of the whole body: when this is the case, take bitters of camomile and orange peels, steeped in boiling water; they may be used a few, gradually increasing their strength ; then take the rustiest iron you can get and put a good chance to a gallon of strong apple cider, and boil it down to a quart; when it begins to boil put in a handful of pine buds, let it cool and put in the white of three eggs, and nine star roots, and take a table spoonful three times a day ; and fiteen drops of laudanum on going to bed, and live on light diet; and if there is nothing more than what you call a common cold, she will be restored to her usual health.

THE OBSTRUCTION OF THE MENSES CONTINUED.

In this distinction, there is a mixed state of the disease; it is the consequence of debility induced by a complaint of some kind, which goes before it; the discharge gradually lessens in quantity; becomes irregular, and at length disappears; and if however the patient declines in a gradual manner, and is subject to dejection of spirits, want of appetite, flashes of heat over the skin, a slight cough, a weakness in the back, coldness of the feet—at times a pressing and bearing down, with a kind of itching and burning in the lower extremities ; and often when the patient makes water it will appear to burn them.   The pains appear to work in the side of some, like pleurisy ; sometimes a tinging in the flesh, like little pins sticking in the patient; a deadness and sleepiness in the flesh, &c.   The remedies must be given to the patient with care, and beware of taking cold.   Except the patient is restored to her common health with care, it will turn to a deep con- sumption, or some fatal complaint.   I have known the severest convulsive fits occasioned by it.

Beat some puccoon roots fine, put a good large table spoonful of sweet fennel seed, the same of dried birch bark—add these ingredients to a quart of apple cider' and let it stand three or four days—for a dose take a table spoonful night and morning, and beware of eat- ing hog-meat or milk, but such as beef, mutton, chicken, squirrels and butter.   If the above medicine should make the patient weak and feeble, when first taken, with sickness at the stomach ; when this subsides, the patient will probably have a craving appetite, but do not eat too much, but eat little and often, and take care of taking cold.   If the medicine makes the pa- tient sick, it is of good effect ; and no doubt will re- store the patient's health.   I have cured many by this medicine.   Again you may get a handful of sweet modly, the same of butterfly roots, and two or three table spoonfuls of camomile flowers, a handful of ver- vine roots, the same of red centaury, put these articles in a quart of rye whisky, and take of this three or four times a day, let your diet be light, beware of getting cold, let your drink be cooling, such as balm tea, cinque- foil, ground-ivy, are also good—if a sweat is necessa- ry, use the tincture of cayenne pepper and gum-myrrh. Take a handful of dried bore-hound, some ginseng root. camomile flowers and orange peels, and the rust of iron, put these in a quart of liquor, shake it well once or twice a day, it is then fit for use. The patient may take half a table spoonful two or three times a day.— This is a medicine which the Indians use in all cases of this kind.

IMMODERATE MENSES.

When the menses continue too long, or come on too often for the strength of the patient, they are said to be immoderate; this most frequently happens to women of a soft delicate habit, to such as use tea and coffee too freely, and who do not take sfficient exercise.— It is sometimes brought on by excessive fatigue; and this may happen to temperate and industrious women. In either case its approach may be known by a pain in the loins and hips; observe this symptom carefully, and on its first appearance let a little blood from the arm; and it will generally prevent the attack for that time. But for the entire removal of it, observe the following directions: So soon as it is known that this complaint is formed, it will be proper to bleed a little from the arm: there are but few instances in which this might not be proper, in greater or lesser quantities. If excessive labor brought on the disease, rest comes in as an essential remedy; cool air is highly proper; this may be applied by placing the patient in such a situation that a current from a door or window may blow upon her; cloths wet in cold vinegar and water may be applied all over the groins. &c., to be changed as they become warm: cold flour in a large quantity applied to the parts, has sometimes succeeded in dangerous cases; cool drinks, as the decoction of nettle roots, or of the greater comfrey, &c. If all these fail, repeat the bleeding: where too strong a motion of the arteries can be ascertained as the cause, it may be generally removed by gentle bleeding, and purging occasionally

repeated. If much weakness, paleness and a disposition to bloat, give half a grain of opium every six hours,
and at intervals of three or four hours, give twelve or
fifteen grains of an equal mixture of alum and gum
kino; nauseate the stomach with small doses from one
to five grains of ipecacuanha; apply blisters to the
wrists and ancles alternately, in all delicate cases; after the removal of the disease for the time being, having recourse to cold bath, exercise, friction with a flesh
brush or flannel, till her health is confirmed.

FLOUR ALBUS OR WHITES.

When a discharge of whitish matter flows instead of
the menses it is called the flour albus or whites; if it
be of a long standing it sometimes assumes a granish
or yellow complection ; becomes acid, sharp and corroding ; and is highly offensive to the smell. When
it happens to young women, it is in most cases a local
disease—I mean by this, that it is never brought on by
any general affection of the system, but is wholly confined to the parts which are its seat, indeed it is sometimes
the case that the menses are discharged entirely in this
way. For the cure, take the rust of iron prepred, one
ounce of gum myrrh, one ounce of nutmeg no. 2, or
cinnamon half an ounce, the whole to be finely
powdered carefully mixed and kept in a close vessel :
if rust of iron cannot be had, the salt of steel will answer, (using half the quantity) of this preparation,
may be taken, from four to six times a day ; if prepared with the salt of steel, four to six grains will be the
dose ; the portion of either ought to be varied according to circumstances, if it excite a little sickness of the
stomach, but if puking or too violent sickness take place
the dose may be lessened; on the other hand if no
considerable effects are observed, it may be enlarged
&c., or take the bark of service tree and make a tea

for your drink ; this is wonderful ; or steep rosin and brimstone in spirits and drink as a bitter; or boil pine buds for tea, or the roots of pine, or what is better turpentine in its soft state mixed with equal quantity of honey, of this mixture a tea spoonful may be taken three times a day ; or for those who can procure it, balsam copaiba, twenty drops in a little new milk three times a day, frequently clense the parts with milk and water. Sometimes an injection made of sixty grains of white vitriol, dissolved in a pint of spring or rain water ; and thrown into the passage by the help of a syringe, three or four times a day, is a most effectual remedy, or bluestone dissolved in old brandy, and used the same way ; and lastly, if ulcers attend, give two or three grains of calomel every third night, and touch the ulcers with a little murcurial ointment, or with an ointment of white or red precipitate of mercury.

Here it might be well to observe that a disease in some degree similar to the flour albus, or more com- monly of a mixed kind, between this and immoderate menses is sometimes the effect of a polypus or excres- cence from the inner surface of the womb. If, there- fore, the discharge should continue after using the pro- per remedies, a polypus ought to be suspected, and a physician or surgeon should be called in to your aid.

A CESSATION OF THE MENSES.

The period of life at which menstruation ccease is always a very critical one to women, as the constitution then undergoes a very considerable change, and it not unfrequently happens, that chronic complaints then arise, which create much disturbance, and, after a time terminate fatally, if not counteracted. The menses seldom ceases all at once, but for some time before their stoppage becomes somewhat irregular, both as to periods and the quantity. When they happen to dissappear suddenly in women of a full plethoric habibit, such persons should be careful to confine themselves to a more pure diet than usual. They should likewise take regular exercise, and keep their body open by a use of some mild laxative, such as senna and manna, if it sho'd not be found sufficiently poweiful, the patient may add a little quinine and jalap, to the same preparation, when the patient is sensible, a seeming fullnes of the vessels, with giddiness and and occasional pains in the head, small bleedings is necessary, if ulcers break out in the legs, or any other part of the body, on a total cessation of the menses, they ought to be regarded as critical discharges, and should by no means be healed up, without substituting some other drain by an issue, should any scirrhous affection of the uterus, take place on a stoppage of the meustrual flux as sometimes happen, all that can be done in such a case is to have recourse to palliatives, such as opium hyoscyamus, and conium, in the manner pointed out in the succeeding disease.

THE DISEASES OF PREGNANCY.

Three different stages evidently exist during a state of pregnancy, each of which have a distinct set of symptoms ; and when we reflect on the alteration which the constitution suffers in consequence of impregnation, and the vast distention and dislodgment of the uterus which prevails at a more advanced period, we cannot be surprised at the complaints and irregularities which then arise. The first stage of pregnancy is usually accompanied with a suppression of the menses, together with fiequent nausea, and vomitting, heart-burn indigestion, peculiar longings, head-ache, giddiness, tooth-ache, and sometimes a slight cough ; the breasts become enlarged, shooting pains extend through them, and the circle round the nipple alters to a dark brown color. There often occurs likewise a feverish disposi-

tion, , with debility, emaciation, irritability, and pe-
vishness of temper, and total alteration of the countenance, every feature of which becomes much sharpened.
Some women breed so easily as to experience hardly
any kind of inconvenice whatever ; whilst others again
are frequently incapable of retaining the least thing on
their stomach, and are thereby reduced to a state of
extreme weakness.

With some women, the vomiting will continue during the whole or greater part of the second stage of
pregnancy, as well as the first ; but this does not usually happen. Partial suppression of urine, with a frequent inclination to void it ; itching about the external
parts of generation, costiveness, tenesmus, and the
piles, are what they are chiefly incommoded by, during
this period. Most women qnicken about the sixteenth
week after conception, at which time the mother be_
comes sensible of the slight efforts of the child ;and
besides the complaints just enumerated, she will then
be liable to sudden faintings, and slight hysteric affections, and extreme weakness.

According to the common received opinion, quickening so termed, has been generally understood to commence at the time when particular sensations are perceived by the mother, supposed to be occasioned by
the first motion of the child. The most usual time of
feeling any such symptoms, is about the latter end of
the fourth, or beginning of the fifth month of pregnancy; at this period the uterus filling up, the pelvis slips
out, and rises above the rim, and from that sudden
transition, women of a delicate constitution and irritable fibre, are apt to faint, more particularly so, if in an
erect position. During the last three months, or third
stage of pregnancy, general uneasiness, restlessness,
costivness, ocdematous swellings of the feet, ancles and
private parts, cramps in the legs and thighs, difficulty of
retaining the urine for any length of time, varicose
swellings of the veins of the belly and lower extremi-

ties, and the piles, are the affections which usually prove most troublesome. In weak delicate women of an irritable habit, convulsive fits sometimes arise which are ever to be regarded in a dangerous light. Nausea and vomiting. It has been observed, that frequent nausea and vomiting are apt to prove somewhat troublesome to pregnant women, and in many cases to reduce them to a state of very great debility. As these most frequently arise immediately upon first getting out of bed in the morning, the patient should be recommended under such circumstances, never to rise until she has taken either a dish of tea, coffee, or whatever else she has usually accustomed herself to for breakfast. If the vomiting should become at any time so severe as to threaten to bring on a miscarriage, for the violence of straining, it may then be advisable to direct two or three table spoonfuls of the saline medicine, to be taken every now and then, in such a manner as that the effervescence shall ensue after it is swallowed; besides which the patient's body should be kept open with some gentle laxative. If these means do not succeed, we may order about six ounces of blood to be drawn from the arm, and which, if necessary, may be repeated in a week's time. The sickness, in such cases, depends on irritation, and is only to be removed with certainty by bleeding. Local applications have been recommended, to abate excessive vomiting. As such, a piece of folded linen cloth, moistened with the tincture of opium, may be kept constantly applied to the region of the stomach. Probably a small addition of ether might increase its good effects. It sometimes happens that vomiting is incessant for many days together, accompanied with great prostration of strength, and constant thirst, and at the same time an utter impossibility of retaining any thing on the stomach. In this state the application of a small blister-plaster to the pit of it, and a constant attention to suffer nothing to be swallowed that can irritate, allowing the patient only new sweet milk, and that by single spoonfuls, have been found to afford relief.

If a considerable degree of nausea prevails, without the ability of throwing up, fourteen or fifteen grains of pulverised ipecacuanha, may then be given, experience having proved that gentle emetic's may be administered with perfect safety to pregnant women. Head ache with plethora. When either head-ache, drowsiness, or a sense of fullness in the vessels, proves troublesome, drawing off a few ounces of blood from the arm in robust women, will most likely be attended with advantage. In those of a weak, irritable, habit, the application of a blister-plaster; one to each temple will be more advisable than bleeding from the system, where the head ache, proves obstinate and resists the other means we have employed. The bowels are at the same time to be kept in a proper state by some gentle aperient. Tooth ache — For the alleviation of the tooth ache, the external as well as internal application of a few drops of the oil of cloves, cajaput, juniper, or any other essential oil, will often prove effectual. Heart burn — If the patient is incommoded by heart burn, half a drachm of magnesia may be taken morning and evening, and if that fails, you may have recourse to charcoal, or globular salts, this is efficacious for the removal of this distressing symptom in pregnant women.

Longings — When pepculiar longings arise in a state of pregnancy, they should always be gratified if possible, as women are apt to miscarry from the axiety these occasion, when not indulged in them; but that the child in the uterus can be marked by any depraved appetite of the mother, be mutilated by any disagreeable object being presented to her, cannot be admittad. All aberrations from the usual form ought to be ascribed to the irregular operation of the powers concerned in generation, and are not produced by the imagination of the mother.

Hysteria — Should any hysterical affection or sudden fainting arise, little more will be necessary than to expose the patient to a free open air, to place her in a horizontal position; and give a glass of cold water with a few drops of the liquor volat, Cornu corvina, or a little wine sufficiently dilutated. Costiveness, piles, &c. Costiveness, partial suppression of urine, and the piles which attend on the second stage of pregnancy are occasioned by the great pressure of the uterus on the rectum and bladder. The first and last of these symptoms are to be obviated by a daily use of some laxative, such as a solution of manna, senna, &c. &c. If necessary a little of the tincture of opium may be added. Itchings — Where a severe itching about the parts of generation attends on pregnancy, it will be proper to keep the woman's body perfectly open with some cooling laxative and to wash the parts three or four times a day, with a diluted solution of lead; such as the vinegar of squills; if such inflammation accompanies the itching, topical bleeding may be requisite. Swellings — The swellings of the feet, ancles and private parts, which arise in the last stage of pregnancy, are occasioned by the pressure made by the womb, which now prevents the free return of the blood from the lower extremities. Gravid women are usually free from these complaints in the morning, but towards night they frequently suffer much from them. Slight scarifications with the edge of a lancet, to discharge the stagnated fluid, with the after application of flannels wrung out in warm infusion of emollient herbs; have been employed in cases of great distention. In general. however, it will only be necessary that the patient does not keep her feet in a pendent position for any length of time. Cramp — Cramp of the legs and thighs are to be relieved by rubbing the parts with cool vinegar, with camphor dissolved in oil, or the liniments here advised, the person wearing stockings in bed. At

9

an advanced period of pregnancy, they are only to
be relieved by labor removing the cause. Where the
stomach is affected with spasms, proper doses of ether
and tincture of opium, with the other means advised
under the head of Hysteria, in cramps of that origin,
will afford the greatest benefit. In such cases, the patient must carefully avoid every kind of food that is
apt to prove flatulent hard of digestion, and she must
keep her body perfectly open.

False pains--Pain somewhat resembling those of labor, and known by the name of false pains, are apt to
come on in an advanced stage of pregnancy, and often
to occason an unnecessary alarm. In such cases, confinement, in a horizontal position, bleeding, if plethoric,
laxative medicines, if costive, and administering small
and frequent doses of some opiate until the patient finds
ease, will be necessary.

Of Convulsions—Cases of puerperal convulsion bear
some likeness to epileptic fits, and it is only by being
aware of the different degree of violence attending
each, that at first sight we can distinguish them. A
fit of puerperal convulsion, is much more severe than
one of epilepsy, and a paroxysm of the former is usually so violent that a woman, who when in health,
was by no means strong, has been so convulsed as to
shake the whole room, and to resist the coercive powers of many attendants. No force can restrain a woman when in these convulsions. The distortion of her
countenance is beyond conception ; in regard to deformity of countenance, nothing bears any resemblance
to the progress of this disease ; the rapidity with
which the eyes open and shut, and the sudden twir-
lings of the mouth, are inconceivable and frightful.

After the first bleeding, the head should be immediately
shaved and a blister of considerable size be applied to
it. The next point to be attended to is to get the bowels to act as quickly as possible, and this will be effected
by throwing up a solution of soft soap as a clyster,

and then giving a strong solution of some neutral salts, as magnesia sulphas, polassae, tartars, or soda with an iufusion of senna.

The warm bath is strongly recommended, among the means for preventing convlusions in women previous to, or during their confinement.

The patient may also be relieved from that state of irritation immediately preceding the convulsou, by dipping feathers in cold water, and dashing it with force over the woman's face as this rouses her, and interrupts the progress of the fit. Where the further application of cold may be deemed necessary and appear advisable, we may throw water over the patient's head bringing this over the side of the bed, and holding an empty pail underneath to receive it. It should be done on the approach of the fit, which may be ascertained by attending to the vibrations of the intercostal muscles. In all cases of puerperal convulsions, after having paid due attention to the lessning of the cause, which has given rise to it, we should uniformly exert our best endeavors to deliver the woman as expeditiously as possible where it is practicable, without violence. When we find that the os-uteri begins to relax and open, and which may take place although there be no labor pain, we must introduce the hand slowly, dilate it, and deliver the child, when convulsions continue after the nuterus is emptied of its contents, all that can be done, is to keep the brain unloaded, the bowels open and the irratibility of the system concentrated by opium, joined with other anti-spasmodics ; such as musk and ether, where the disorder continues many hours the patient should have a large blister applied to the head and if a benefit is not obtained in twenty four hours, one may also be applied to the inside of each leg. These by exciting an irration upon a part distant from the disease, may tend to diminish the diseased action, and thereby afford some relief.

To prevent puerperal convulsions from supervening

as they are in every instance to be considered as highly dangerous ; particularly at an advanced stage of
pregnancy. It will be prudent in robust and plethoric
habits, to pay an early attention to a use of the lancet,
during the progress of pregnancy, by drawing off a
quantity of blood at different periods, taking care at
the same time, and particularly near the termination
of pregnancy, to keep the bowels open by cooling purgatives. In women of irritable constitution, all exciting
causes should be carefully avoided and the habit be
strengthened as much as possible, and thereby be rendered less susceptible of disagreeable or ready impressions.

ON THE PRACTICE OF MIDWIFERY.

I consider this a practice of great importance, and
shall therefore set down a few instructions respecting
the proper course that should be pursued in time
of labor. I shall use the plainest lauguage possible
in treating on this subject so that the midwife may
have a thorough knowledge of the performance and
treatment of midwifery.

The abdomen is the name given to the belly ; it is
the soft covering of the bowels, extending from the
breast down to the following bone, which is called the
pubis : This bone stands forwards, forming an arch between the hips, and is called by some the bearing bone.
It has a peculiar kind of joints in the middle, which
sometimes opens in case of difficult labor, and when
this happens, it is commonly followed by a collection
of matter, which is distresing to the last degree, very
difficult to cure, and sometimes fatal to the patient.—
The sacrum is the part of the bones which is fixed between the hips backwards, and is opposite to the pubis.
The sacrum extends itself downwards and forwards,
forming a curve, and makes it necessary to regulate the
passage of the child in a corresponding direction. The

large passage or cavity, made by these two bones. together with the othe1 bones of the hips, is called the
pelvis. If this cavity is much less than the common,
or out of shape, so as to prevent the passage of ·the
child, the pelvis is said to be distorted ; this distortion
may be effected several ways. The common distance
between the sacrum and pelvis, is rather more than
four inches, but it is sometimes found to be no more
than one. The lower part of the sacrum, which bends
forwards and inwards, forming a curve as above, in
young women, admits of a little motion backwards,
so as to make the passage of the child more easy.—
But in some instances especially in those women who
do not marry till they become old maids, it is so strong
as not to admit of any motion at all. In addition to this,
it sometimes bends so far inwards, as very much to obstruct the passage. The mons-veneris is the fatty
substance which covers the pubis, and extends downwards and sidewards towards the two groins. The
Labia, the two thick soft pieces of skin which passes
on either side, still downwards from the mons-veneris,
the pudendum, external parts of generation ; of these
the labia are the principal parts. The perinacum, the
parts which begins at the lower angel of the 'labia, and
extends backwarks to the anus or fundament. This is
subject to be torn in child bearing. The vaginian, or
passage from the pudendum to the womb, (the uterius,
the name of the womb) at the upper end of the vagina
is an opening into the womb, called the os-uteri, or the
mouth of the womb, (the placenta) the after birth,
called also the cake ; and with the membranes, in-
cluding the child waters, &c., is sometimes called the
secundines, the umbilical cord, the navel string, the
fœtus, the child while in the womb. These names, I
will add in this place the five following terms, expressive of certain changes which takes place in the act of
child bearing ; Parturation—The act of bringing forth
a child ; is another name for labour.

Dilation—The act of stretching and opening at the same time. This is applied to os-uteri, and to the pudendum. Distention—The act of stretching or making more open. Expel—The act of turning out.—This is performed by the uterus, when it contracts which it endeavors to do by certain periodical exertions, called pains.

Presentation—The act of precenting. This term is applied to the position of the child, and particularly to the part of the child which is first sensible to the touch at the mouth of the womb when labor is coming on.—There is the names of the different parts of generation; and again, the common time for complete gestation, is forty weeks; at the expiration of which the process of labor commences, every labor should be called natural, if the head of the child is present. If the labor be completed within twenty-four hours, if no artificial aid be required, if the labor be prolonged beyond twenty-four hours, it may be called difficult, &c.

SYMPTOMS OF PRESENT LABOR.

The first symptoms of present labor, is an anxiety arising from a dread of danger, or doubt of safety.—This anxiety will be increased if the patient should have heard of accidents or deaths, in any late or similar case. It is the duty of the midwife to soothe and comfort her when in this situation, by suitable language, and a diligent attention to every complaint. But in the mean time, she should by no means be persuaded to offer assistance before it is necessary. At the commencement of labor, women have commonly one or more chills, or fits of shivering, with or without a sense of cold. But should there be one strong and distinct chill or shivering fit, it may be a dangerous symptom. There will be some difficulty in voiding the urine; it should therefore be evacuated frequently, otherwise it may ultimately become necessary to introduce a ca-ther. There will sometimes be a frequent painful dis-position to go to stool ; this ought to be considered a favorable symptom. A glyster or two prepared of milk and water, or thin gruel, may serve to correct the pain; or if no such disposition be present, the glysters may serve to evacuate the bowels artificially. The mucous discharge which before was without color, will after the commencement of labor, be tinged with blood; this appearance is commonly called the shew. If to-gether with the above symptoms; the usual pains be present, the presumption is very strongly in favor of approaching parturition.

COMMON APPEARANCE OF TRUE PAINS

First.—The true pains usually begin in the loins or lower part of the back, pass round into the abdomen and end at the pubis, or upper part of the thighs.—Sometimes, however, they take the opposite direction, that is, beginning at the thighs or pubis, and ending in the loins ; sometimes too, they are confined to one par-ticular spot, as the back, abdomen, thighs, and even to the knees, heels or feet, and in some instances, other parts are affected, the stomach, head, &c. Second.—the true labor pains are periodical, with intervals of twenty, fifteen, ten or five minutes, and moderate pains frequently repeated, are safer than more severe ones at greater intervals. An experienced midwife may gen-erally judge of the nature of present pains from the tone of the patient's voice. The first change affected by the pains, consists in a dilatation of the parts. For-cible and quick distention, gives a sensation like that produced by the infliction of a wound : and the tone of voice will be in a similar manner interrupted and shrill, these are vulgarly called cutting, grinding or rending pains. When the internal parts ar sufficiently opened, the child begins to descend, and then the patient is by her feelings obliged to make an effort to expel, and the expression will be made with a continued and grave tone of voice; or she will hold her breath and be silent: these are called bearing pains. It is a common thing to say that women have fruitless pains; this is an unfair and discouraging statement. No person in labor ever had a pain depending on her labor which was in vain. In the beginning, pains are usually slight in their degree, and have long intervals. But as the labor advances, they become more violent, and the intervals are shorter. Sometimes the pains are alternately stronger; the next weaker, or one stronger and two weaker; but every variety, has its own peculiar advantage, being wisely adapted to the state of the patient. Nothing therefore, can be more preposterous, than any kind of artificial attempt to add to the strength of the pains, or to hasten their return. It is wrong even to direct the patient to help herself. The supposed skill of midwives, in these points, has done more mischief to society, than the most skilful practice ever did good, &c. Though false pains may be detected and removed, a case may occur when it may be necessary to determine whether present pains be true or false; because if false pains be encouraged or permitted to continue, they may at length occasion premature labor. Then some known cause commonly goes before and brings on false pains, as fatigue of any kind, especially too long standing on the feet, sudden and violent motion of the body, great costiveness, a diarrhœa, a general feverish disposition, some violent agitation of the mind, or the like. But the most certain way for detecting false pains, is by an actual examination; this operation is commonly called taking a pain. The position in which women are placed when it is necessary to examine them, varies in different countries, and indeed, almost every midwife has her own opinion; but most regular men direct the women to repose on a

couch or bed upon her left side, with her knees bent
and drawn up towards the abdomen ; and this is certainly the most convenient and decent method. The
examination should be performed with the utmost care,
decency and tenderness. If there be perceptible pressure on the os-uteri, or if it be perceived to dilate during the coutinuance of a pain, the woman may be considered as really in labor ; but if neither pressure nor
dilation can be felt, the conclusion may be drawn, that
the pains are false. If it be determined that the pains
are false, it will be proper to attempt to remove them ;
when occasioned by fatigue of any kind, the patient
should rest in bed ; if she be of a feverish disposition,
she should lose some blood. Generally it will be proper to give a dose or two of manna with sweet oil, or
castor oil, or the like ; mild and opening glysters should
be injected every three or four hours till the bowels
are emptied. After these evacuations, which should be
repeated according to the exigency of the case, she
should have a grain of opium, with one grain of ipecacuanha every three hours, till she be composed. Let it
be observed, however, that an examination should never
be made in too great haste; and if it be probable that the
patient is really in labor, an examination ought to be made
until the membranes are broken, or till the os-uteri is fully
dilated; but more of this will be given in another place.

PROGRESS OF NATURAL LABOR.

There may be said to be three stages, in the progress
of natural labor. The first includes all the circumstances of the pains of the complete dilatation of the os-uteri,
the breaking of the membranes, and the discharge of
the waters. The second includes those which occur
at the time of the opening of the os-uteri to the expulsion of the child ; and the third, includes all the circumstances which relate to the separation and exclusion of
the placenta. But to treat of each of these stages,

more particularly, and in order: The os-uteri is not always found in the same central position; nor does it always dilate in the same length of time. The first part of the dilatation is generally made very slowly; but when the membranes containing the waters begin to insinuate themselves, they act like a wedge, and the operation proceeds much more rapidly. It cannot well be told with certainty, how long time will be required in any case for the complete dilatation of the os-uteri, yet some conjecture may be made. If, for example, after the pains have continued three hours, the os-uteri should be dilated to the size of one inch; and three hours more will be required for a complete dilation; making in all eight hours. This calculation supposes the labor to go on regularly, and with equal strength. But the os-uteri sometimes remains for hours in the same state, and yet when it begins to dilate, the complete dilatation is soon perfected. Again, in some cases the dilatation proceeds on regularly for a while, and then is suspended for many hours, and afterwards returns with great rigor. With first children, this stage is commonly tedious and very painful; some considerable judgment is therefore necessary on the part of the mid-wife, for supporting the patient and confidence of the suffering woman, as the labor proceeds, the pains becomes more frequent and forcible. If the dilatation should take place, with difficulty, there will sometimes be sickness of the stomach and vomiting, this is a favorable circumstance, as it commonly has a tendency to relax the system; at length, after a greater or lesser number of hours as the case may be, the dilatation is effected. But let it be carefully observed, that no artificial aid is to offered during this part of the process. It may indeed be well enough to pretend to assist, with the intention to compose the mind of the patient, and inspire her with confidence. But be assured, that all manuel interposition will retard the progress of the dilatation, let the patient and by standers be importunate; pain on the one hand and ignorance on the other may excuse them. But the midwife must be firm in discharge of her duty; care must be taken not to break the membranes, should an examination be deemed necessary when the os-uteri is fully dilated; they are usually broken by the force of pains. If this should not be the case, they will protrude outward, in the form of a bag, and then are of no further use. If the labor has not been disturbed, the child is common-ly born speedily after the natural rupture of the mem-branes: and therefore, if the birth be delayed after this event takes place, it will be a very proper time to make a careful examination of the state of things. Here I must be permitted to remark, that touching the parts too frequently, is highly pernicious; the juices furnish-ed by nature for moistening, softening, and by these means preparing the parts for distention must be im-properly exhausted by repeated applications of the hand; If the passage be thus left dry, it will be much disposed to irritation, and the whole process may be deranged.

In every difficult case which has come under my ob-servation, I have been able to trace all the existing evils back to the common error, of too early taking in hand, as the operation is commonly called. Your pomatums, oils. lead, and ointments, are poor substitutes for natur-al fluids, which are wiped away. Indeed they may do· injury by clogging the mouths of little vessels through which these fluids are secreted; by escaping any such injury it happens pretty commonly that women taken at surprise have better times, than when aided by good midwives of the neighborhood; if there be no irregu-larity, nature is always competent to the task appoint-ed her of God; and the only circumstance which can make it necessary to call in a widwife at all, are a pos-sibility of such irregularity, and the convenience of having her dexterity in the management of the placen-ta, dressing the child, &c.

SECOND STAGE OF NATURAL LABOR.

The second stage of labor includes all circumstances attending the descent of the child through the pelvis, the dilatation of the external parts, and the final expulsion of the child.   In general it will follow that the further the labor is advanced before the discharge of the waters the more safely will this second stage be accomplished; as the head passes through the pelvis, it undergoes various changes of position, by which it is adapted to the form of each part of the passage, and that more or less, readily, according to the size of the head, strength of the pains, &c. Whether those changes are produced quickly or in a tedious manner; whether in one or more hours, it can by no means be proper to interfere, for the powers of the constitution will produce their proper effect with less injury and more propriety than the most dexterous midwife. When the head begins to press upon the external part first, every pain may be suffered to have its full and natural effect. But when part of the head is fully exposed and the fore part of the perinaeum is on the stretch, it is necessary to use some precaution to prevent it from being torn, and the more expeditious the labor, the more is this caution necessary. Some have thought that if the external parts be very rigid they should be frequenty anointed with some kind of ointment; nothing can equal the natural juices. But if from any cause, the parts become heated and dry, flannels wrung out of warm water, should be applied for some time, and afterwards some very mild ointments might not be amiss. Women with first children are most subject to inconvenience and difficulty in these respects: to prevent any injury of the external parts, the only safe and effectual plan is to retard for a certain time the passage of the head through them; therefore instead of encouraging the patient at this time to use her utmost exertions to hasten the birth, she should be convinced

of its impropriety, and be dissuaded from using any
voluntary exertion. If she cannot be regulated according to your wishes, her efforts must be counteracted
by some equivalent external resistence : this may be
performed by blacing the finger and thumb of the right
hand upon the head of the child, during the time of a
pain ; or by placing the balls of one or both thumbs on
the thin edge of the parinaeum, with first children. If
there be great danger of laceration, the right hand may
be used as before, and the palm of the left hand wound
round with a cloth may be applied over the whole perinaeum where it must be firmly continued during the
violence of the pain. It is proper to proceed in this
way, till the parts are sufficiently dilated ; then the
head may be permitted to slide through them in the
slowest and gentlest manner, paying the strictest attention, till it is perfectly cleared of the perinaeum.
If there should be any difficulty when the perinaeum
slides over the face, the fore finger of the right hand
may be placed under its edge, by which it may be
cleared of its mouth and chin before the support given
by the left hand be withdrawn ; the assistance should
be applied in a proper direction, and with uniformity ;
otherwise the danger of injury to the external parts
will be increased by irregular or partial pressure, the
head being expelled, it is commonly deemed necessary
to extract the body of the child without delay ; but
experience has now taught that there is no danger, and
that is far safer for the mother and the child, to wait for
the return of the pains, and when the shoulders of the
child begin to advance and the external parts are again
brought to the stretch, the same support should be given to the perinaeum as before. The child should
then be conducted in a proper direction, so as to keep
its weight from resting too heavily upon the perinaeum;
two or three pains are sometimes necessary for the expulsion of the shoulders: after the head is born, the
child should be placed in such a situation that the ex-

ternal air may have free access to its mouth; but let
its head be covered.   Having taken the proper care of
the mother, it will be necessary to proceed to the third
and last part of the operation.

THE THIRD STAGE OF NATURAL LABOR — THE MANAGEMENT OF PLACENTA &c.

There is a proper time for dividing the funis or umbilical cord; before the child breathes or cries, a motion of the arteries of the cord may be felt beating like
the pulse; but after it breathes and cries, this pulsation,
or motion ceases, and the string becomes quite relaxed
and soft.   These circumstances ought to take place before the umbilical cord is divided; ten, fifteen, and
sometimes twenty minutes are required for the complete relaxation of the naval string; then let it be tied
in two places, and divided between them, soon after
the birth of the child, and whether the womb contracts
in a favorable manner to the separation of the cake.
Most women are extremely uneasy till the placenta is
removed, and suppose the sooner it is removed the better; but this uneasiness is unnecessary, and all hurry
is improper.   After the birth of the child, let the first
attention be paid to the mother; tranquility should be
restored to her mind, and the hurried circulation of the
blood should be calmed; she should be recovered from
her fatigue, and her natural state regained as soon as
possible.   With this design, let her be kept quiet, af-
fording her at the same time some suitable refreshment.
In the course of ten, fifteen, or twenty minutes, the
pains will return for the purpose of expelling the placenta, and it will be expelled without any kind of artificial aid, which should never be employed when it can
be avoided; but if it descends too slowly, the midwife
may take hold of the cord, and by pulling in a gentle
manner, and in a proper direction, may afford some

assistance — and this should be done only in time of pain. After the cake is brought down into the vagina, whether by the natural pains, or with the artificial aid as above, it must be suffered to remain there till excluded by the pains; this may prevent a dangerous flooding, if an hour be requisite for the exclusion. After it enters the vagina, no assistance ought to be offered, but after that time, it may again be gently pulled in time of pains. No objection should be raised to this plan, from any supposed advantage to be derived to the child, from laying the cake upon its belly, on the hot embers, in hot wine, and the like; all this is of little account, Let it then be a settled point that hurry is improper, either in dividing the string or removing the cake. Haste in the first may destroy the child, in the last must injure the mother in a greater or less degree; if the ill effects be not immediately perceived, she will at length be sensible of the injury, when her health gradually declines. The conclusion to be drawn from the foregoing is, that parturation is a natural process of the constitution which generally needs no assistance; and when it is natural, it should always be suffered to have its own course without interruption, &c.

INTRODUCTION TO DIFFICULT LABOR.

In consequence of their natural construction the women must be subject to greater pain and difficulty in parturation. Yet, by the peculiar form of the mother, and the original construction of the head of the child, ample provision is made for overcoming the difficulties to which they are subject. But by the customs of society, and various other causes, women are rendered subject to diseases and accidents which increase their natural inconveniences, and produce new causes of danger. Therefore there will be occasions which will require assistance. The first distinction of labor re-

quiring assistance of art, may be called difficult, and
every labor in which the head of the child presents,
but which is delayed longer than twenty-four hours,
ought to be classed under this head ; difficult or tedious
labors may be of four kinds ; those which are rendered
difficult from a too weak or an irregular action of the
womb. Those which are occasioned by a certain rigidity or firmness of the parts, in consequence of which
dilatation is tedious and difficult; those in which a
quick and easy passage of the child is prevented by
some distortion of the pelvis, or too large a size of the
head; those of the soft parts which are reduced difficult from diseases.

FIRST KIND OR DIFFICULT LABOR.

The action of the womb is sometimes too weak, in
consequence of great distention. In a case of this
sort, the safest, and frequently the only remedy, is to
allow the patient sufficent time to walk or stand, pursue any amusement, or choose that position which she
may prefer. Sometimes, however, frequent glysters of
warm milk and water, or thin gruel, might be injected;
or if the pains should be feeble, and come on in a very
slow manner, and if the labor be far advanced, it will
be proper to give a glyster of gruel made more vivita-
ting, by the addition of an ounce of common table salt,
or a like quantity of purging salt, whichever may be
most convenient. The action of the womb may be
feeble and tedious, in consequence of being partial or
incomplete; in a case of this kind, the patient will com-
plain that the child lies high in the stomach ; or she
will have cramp like pains in various parts of the abdomen, which seem quite ineffectual ; if these pains be
great and different from common labor pains, they are
commonly the effect of a feverish disposition ; and if
so, the patient may loose some small quantities of blood:

she may take thirty or forty drops of spirits of nitre, in a cup of some kind of cooling tea, every two or three hours.

Her bowels must be kept open with glysters, or gentle doses of manna, castor-oil or purging salts; and sometimes it will be found useful to anoint the whole abdomen with warm oil; if little fever be present, she might walk about the room in the intervals between the pains. If she should have suffered long, after the blood letting and a glyster or two, she should take forty-five or fifty drops of opium mixed with one and a half grains of ipecacuanha, to be repeated if necessary at the end of six hours; the powder is preferable to the tincture of opium. In this case, sometimes the pains are not sufficiently strong to break the membranes containing the waters. If the presumption be that the membranes are too ridgid, or if sufficient time may have been allowed, it may become necessary to break them artificially.

But as was observed under the head of natural labors, this must be done with the greatest caution. It should be first known, that the os-uteri is fully dilated, and care must be taken not to be deceived in this point, because the os-uteri is sometimes so thinly and uniformly spread over the head of the child before it is in any degree dilated, as very much to resemble the membranes. If it be determined to break the membranes, no instrument is necessary but the finger, or at most the finger nail prepared for the purpose, by being cut and turned up; the shortness of the funis, or umbilical cord, may be the cause of difficult babor, resembling that which is the effect of a feeble action of the womb. It may therefore be explained in this place. The umbilical cord may be short originally, or may be rendered so by being wound round the neck, body, or limbs of the child. If the child should be drawn back upon the declension of a pain, the shortness of the umbilical cord

10

may be always suspected ; by allowing sufficient time, this inconvenience will commonly be overcome. If however, the child should not be born, after waiting long enough, it may be necessary to change the position of the patient, and instead of reposing on a bed or couch, as advised in the instructions for taking a pain, she may be placed upon the lap of one of the assistants; it will be frequently found advantageous to prefer this position in lingering cases, especially when the parts seem fully prepared for dilation, when the head of the child is expelled, the funis may be brought forwards over the head, or backwards over the shoulders; but if neither can be done, it may be necessary to wait for the effect of time, it is not so dangerous as some suppose for the child to remain sometime in this position; but the air should have free access to its mouth. But when it can no longer be considered safe, the funis must be divided, with the usual precaution of tying, &c.— If the child should be dead and swelled, the labor will commonly be difficult, and put on appearances similar to those of the foregoing cases: it may be found necessary in an instance of this sort, to place a towel or handkerchief round the neck of the child, and then by taking hold of both ends, considerable aid may be afforded.— But if this method should not succeed, one or both arms should be brought down, and included in the handkerchief, by which means still greater force may be applied. In all cases, however, where it can be done with safety, it will be more safe and humane, to wait the effect of natural efforts than to use much force.— Consumption and other diseases, with general debility, commonly causes great apprehensions, about the issue of parturition. But if there be no untoward circum-stances in the way, it will be found that there is a pecu-liar balance obtaining between the strength of the pa-tient, and the disposition of the parts concerned for dilation ; give them time and they will be delivered.— When labor is common, there is generally a sense of heat, quickness of the pulse, thirst, flushed cheeks, in one word a general fever, sick disposition; these appearances may be considered natural efforts for carrying on the depending operation of the system; but the fever runs sometimes too high, and exhausts those powers of the system which ought to have been otherwise applied. When this is the case, nothing can be more erroneous than the common and almost universal plan of giving wine spirits, or other cordials. This kind of treatment, is calculated to increase the fever and destroy the pains. Instead of spirits, wine, or opium, have recourse to cooling drinks, and moderate blood letting, to be repeated according to the circumstances; to these may be added frequent mild glysters, and a gentle purge or two, &c. The room should be kept cool and well aired, and the patient should be kept cool and well aired also, and to be composed as much as possible. Fat and inactive women, very frequently have slow and lingering labor, they seem subject to debility of the indirect kind; in every case of this sort, it must be very improper to make use of spirits, &c., to hasten the pains. Patients under the impression of fear, will almost in every instance be subject to a tedious labor; and as the time is prolonged, their fears will naturally increase, so that ultimately they may be brought into danger by their own cowardly imagination. The midwife should therefore use discreet measures to inspire more favorable sentiments, &c. Concerning letting blood in time of labor, it cannot be admissable in every case, even with the most robust women. But if there be fever, or if the pains be very strong, and the exertions of the woman seem vehement, in either of these cases it is necessary to lose blood.

DIFFICULT LABOR.

Most women with their first children suffer more or

less from the difficult distension of the parts concerned in parturiton; but the ridgidity, which is the cause commonly lessens with every child, in proportion to the number she has; and has sufficient resources within herself for delivery—sometimes blood letting is necessary. In this case, if the woman be advanced in age at the time of having her first child, this rigidity of the parts will be the greater, and of course the labor may be more difficult. Women of this distinction or description, might generally avoid much inconvenience by occasional blood letting towards the close of pregnancy, by making frequent use of gentle laxatives, as manna, sweet oil, castor oil and the like, sitting over the steam of water every night at bed time. It may be observed, however, that it frequently happens that women at forty five, fare as well as they could have done with their first child at twenty five; none therefore ought to be discouraged. The natural efforts of the constitution in these cases are astonishing.

After reading these instructions through,
Midwives will see they have much to do ;
To natures call attend with care,
And then you'll have nothing to fear.

You should at least possess the skill,
So that you may your call fulfill ;
In exercises of this kind,
The above instructions strictly mind.

A specific antidote I'll name,
Which will promte or relieve the pain ;
When nature's effort is thus at hand,
To the following recipe attend.

Steep red raspberry leaves a while—
A little cayene may be addedd too,
And let the patient drink the same,
It will relieve, or promote the pain.

LITHASIS, OR THE GRAVEL AND STONE,

These diseases depend upon a peculiar disposition of the fluids, and more particularly the secretion of the kidneys, to form a calculous matter, and have been supposed to be owning to the presence of an acid principle in them, termed the urine acid, which seems confirmed by the benefit derived from a course of alkaline medicine. A long use of fermented liquors, and wine abounding with tartar, may possibly in some constitutions prove occasional causes of gravel and stone.— It has also been long supposed that water impregnated with sulphate and carbonate of lime, constituting what is called hard water, predisposes persons to be afflicted with the gravel and stone ; instances have been adduced where a stone has arisen from the accidental introduction of some substance in the bladder, thereby forming a nucleus. That a morbidly increased secretion of of gravelly matter frequently occurs, independent of external causes, we have the most satisfactory proof in the hereditary disposition of many families to this complaint. The real cause of the formation of calculi remain, however, still unknown. An excess of uric acid is generally supposed to be the proximate one. Those who are in the decline of life, and who have been much engaged in sedentary employments, as likewise those who are much afflicted with the gout, are in general very subject to nephritic complaints ; but it is a matter of notoriety that the period of life from infancy to about fifteen years, is most subject to the formation of calculi in the bladder, and that the children of the poor are afflicted in a greater proportion than those of the opulent. From the difference in the structure of the urinary passages in the sexes, men are much more liable to them than women. In warm climates we seldom meet with instances of calculours concutions forming of any size either in the kidneys or bladder, as the particles of sand deposited from the urine usually pass

off before they can adhere together, owing to the relaxed state of the parts, but in cold ones they are found
frequently of considerable magnitude.   A fit of the
gravel is attend with a fixed pain in the loins, numbness
of the thigh on the side affected, nausea and vomiting,
and not unfrequently with a slight suppression of urine.
As the irritating matter removes from the kidneys down
into the ureter, it sometimes produces such acute
pain as to occasion faintings and convulsive fits.   The
symptoms which attend on a stone in the bladder are a
frequent inclination to make water, which flows in a
small quantity, is often suddenly interrupted, and is a-
voided towards the end with pain in the glans penis.—
The patient, moreover, cannot bear any kind of rough
motion ; neither can he make use of any severe exercise without enduring great torture, and perhaps bringing on either a dischare of bloody urine ; or some degree of temporary suppression.   With these symptoms
he experiences pain in the neck of the bladder, tenesmus
itching and uneasiness in the anus, frequent nausea,
and sometimes a numbness of one or both thighs, with a
retraction of one of the testicles, the treatment, when
you discover the above symptoms you may readily
conclude what is the disease, you will get a peck of
smart weed the same of the tops of wild indigo, boil this
well in two or three gallons of water down to one
quart then strain it add one gill of whiskey, a half pound
of white sugar, of this you will take a table spoonful
three times a day, you will also take twenty drops of
the compound horsemint, three or four times a day in a
little water, look for horsemint in the materia medica,
if in case there should be too free a portion of urine
from the effects of the dose, a less portion should be
taken, if there appears to be much pain about the kidneys take a half a teaspoonful of the tincture of cubebs with ten drops of laudanum three or four times a
day, keep the bowels open with mild purgatives and
nothing more is necessary ; I have relieved hundreds

. of this disease with the above prescription, let the diet be light and cooling.

ST. VITUS' DANCE.

This disease is marked by convulsive actions, most generally confined to one side and affecting principally the arm and leg.   When any motion is attempted to be made, various fibres of the muscles act which ought not, and thus a contrary effect is produced from what the patient intended. It is chiefly incited to young persons of both sexes, but particularly those of a weak constitution, or whose health and vigor have been impaired by confinement, or by the use of scanty and improper nourishment, and makes its attacks between the age of ten to fifteen, occurring but seldom after that of puberty.   By some physicians it has been considered rather as a paralytic affection, than as a convulsive disorder, and has thought to arise from a relaxation of the muscles, which being unable to perform their functions in moving the limbs ; shake them irregular by jerks.   St. Vitus' is occasioned by various irritations, as teething, worms, acid matter in the bowels, offensive smells, poisons, &c.   It arises likewise in consequence of violent affections of the mind, as horror, fright and anger.   In many cases it is produced by general weakness of the system, and irritability of the nervous system, and in a few it takes place from sympathy at seeing the disease in others.   The fits are sometimes preceded by a coldness of the feet and limbs or a kind of tingling sensation, that ascends like cold air up the spine, and there is a flatulent pain in the left side, with obstinate costiveness.   At other times the accession begins with yawning, stretching, anxiety about the heart, palpitations, nausea, difficulty of swallowing, noise in the ears, giddiness, and pains in the head and teeth, and then comes on the convulsive mo-

tions. These discover themsevles at first by a kind of
lameness or instability of one of the legs, which the
peison draws after him in an odd and ridiculous manner as if it was practice, nor can he hold the arm of
the same side still for a moment ; for if he lays it on
his breast, or any other part of his body, it is forced
quickly from thence by an involuntary convulsive motion. If he is desirous of drinking, he uses many sin-
gular gesticulations before he can carry the cup to his
head, and it is forced in various directions, till at length
he gets it to his mouth, when he pours the liquor down
his throat with great haste, as if he meant to afford
amusement to the bystanders. Sometimes various at-
tempts at running and leaping take place, and at others
the head and trunk of the body, are affected with convulsive motions. The eye loses its lustre and intelli-
gence, and the countenance is pale and expressive of
vacancy ; deglutition is occasionally performed with
difficulty, and articulation is often impeded, and sometimes completely suspended. In the advanced periods
of the disease, flaccedity and wasting of the muscular
flesh takes place, the consequence of constant irritation
of abated appetite, and impaired digestion. In many
instances the mind is afflicted with some degree of fatu-
ity, and often shows the same causeless emotions, such
as weeping and laughing, which occur in hysteria.
When this disease arises in children, it usually ceases
again before the age of puberty, and in adults is often
carried off by a change from the former mode of life.
Unless it passes into some other disease, such as epilepsy, or its attacks are violent, it is not attended with
danger. Where chorea arises in those of a weak irritable habit, and is wholly unconnected with any species
of irritation, either of teething, worms, or acrid matter in the first passages, we should not employ evacu-
ants, but have recourse to strengthening remedies, with
the view of increasing the tone of the muscular system. In the treatment of this disease bleed freely—

give purgative medicines, produce a regular action on the nerves, give strengthening tonics, &c. &c.

SUPPRESSION AND DIFFICULTY OF URINE.

When there is a frequent desire of making water, attended with much difficulty in voiding it, the complaint is called dysuria or strangury ; and when there is a total suppression of urine, it is known by the name of ischuria. Both ischuria and dysuria are distinguished into acute, when arising in consequence of inflammation, and chronic, when proceeding from any other cause, such as calculous, &c. The causes which give rise to these diseases are, an inflammation of the urethra, occasioned either by venereal sores, or by a use of acrid injections, inflammation of the veru-montanum, bladder or kidneys, considerable enlargements of the hemorrhoidal veins, a lodgement of indurated fæces in the rectum, spasm at the neck of the bladder, the absorption of cantharides, applied externally or taken internally, excess in drinking either spirituous or vinous liquors, or particles of gravel sticking in the neck of the bladder, or lodging in the urethra, and thereby producing irritation. Gout, by being translated to the neck of the bladder, will sometimes occasion these complaints. In many instances, the obstruction of the flow of urine, is in a great measure, owing to a diseased action of the muscles ; in some of them it is entirely to be attributed to this cause. A very frequent cause however of both dysuria and ischuria is an enlargement, or other diseased state of the prostrate gland, a complaint with which men in advanced life, are very apt to be afflicted. It is usually excited by full living of every kind, inebriety, indulging to excess with women, or producing frequent excitement in the seminal vessels by masturbation, severe attacks of gonorrhea, a confined state

11

of the bowels, and exposed to cold. Indeed, whatever increases the circulation of the blood in these parts beyond the healthy standard, may become a cause of inflammation in this gland, the blood vessels of which, lose their tone in an advanced period of life. From various dissections made by Sir Edward Home, it appears that when the prostrate gland becomes diseased, it is not its body, or lateral portion, which in general are principally enlarged, but its middle lobule, which gradually becoming of an increased size, presses inward towards the cavity of the bladder in the form of a nipple—pushes the internal membrane of the bladder before it, obstructs the flow of urine, and gives to dysuria and tenesmus, with many constitutional symptoms. In dysuria there is a frequent inclination to make water, attended with smarting pain, heat, and difficulty in voiding it, together with a sense of fullness in the region of the bladder.

The symptoms often vary, however, according to the cause which has given rise to it. If it proceeds from a calculous in the kidney or ureter, besides the affections mentioned, it will be accompanied with nausea, vomiting, and acute pains in the loins and region of the ureter and kidney, of the side affected. When the stone in the bladder or gravel in the urethra is the cause, an acute pain will be felt at the end of the penis, particularly on voiding the last drops of urine, and the stream of water will either be divided in two, or be discharged in a twisted manner, not unlike a cork-screw. If an enlargement, or scirrhus of the prostrate gland, has occasioned the suppression or difficulty of urine, a hard indolent tumor unattended with an acute pain may readily be felt in the perinæum, or by introducing the finger in one. Dysuria is seldom attended with much danger, unless by neglect it should terminate in a total obstruction. Ischuria may always be regarded as a dangerous complaint, when it continues for any length of time, from the great distension of the bladder, and other consequent inflammation which ensues. In these cases where neither a bougie nor a catheter can be in-troduced, the event in all probability will be fatal, as few patients will submit to the only means of drawing off the urine, before a considerable degree of inflamma-tion and tendency to gangrene have taken place.— When surprise has arisen in consequence of the appli-cation of a blister, as sometimes happens, nothing more will be necessary than to direct the patient to drink plentifully of warm diulent liquors, such as a thin solu-tion of gum-linseed tea, or barley water. When it proceeds from any other cause, and the symptoms are violent, a strong solution of smart weed, and of horse mint, and parsley, fleebane—(this last see materia med-ica.) These articles should all be put in a vessel, with a sufficiency of water, and boil the same down to a strong decoction and strain it, and let it settle, and pour it off from the sediment, add to this preparation a small quantity of spirits, and use it moderately for your constant drink.

TONIC DECOCTION.

Take half a burdock root, half a spignard root, two ounces seneca snake root, one ounce blood root, four ounces black cherry-tree bark, two ounces prickly ash bark, and a little comfrey root; put water enough to these to cover them well in a kettle and boil two hours and pour off or strain—and should there be more than a quart of the decoction, boil it down to one quart.— Add to this decoction molasses sufficient to keep it from spoiling, let her take about three wine glasses full in a day, early in the morning, at eleven, and on going to bed. Should the bowels need moving, a little physic may be given, as salts or castor-oil. Let her diet be as nutritive as she can digest—should she gain strength so as to be able to ride out, let her do so, taking care not to fatigue her.

WINTER FEVER.

At night, give at dark and at nine o'clock, four grains of calomel and two grains of ipecac, and if that does not nauseate the stomach, give four grains of ipecac with the calomel; if the calomel does not operate well, give pink and senna next morning, as hot as can be drank, every hour, give Dovers' powders, as large doses as the stomach will bear ; if there is much pain in the side, apply a mustard plaster, and if that does not answer put on a large blister, and let it draw a deep blister ; keep the feet warm with any thing that is convenient.

ERYSIPELAS—HOW CURED.

Take three ounces of tobacco, three grains of gum myrrh, and three grains of gum camphor; this is all to be well pulverized, and then well moistened or wet with strong vinegar, and put to the part affected, let this remain on for two hours, then put on another one, after taking off the old one, and so on for three or four times.

TO STOP BLOOD—WARRANTED.

Take rye meal, or some call it rye flour, and brown or parch it in a pan or skillet, and put this powder in the wound, and bind up the part that is wounded. We have never known this to fail of having the desired effect.

AGUE BITTERS.

Take three pounds of dogwood bark, one and a half pounds of poplar bark, three fourth pounds of cherry-tree bark, (all inside barks,) put these barks into five gallons of water, boil it down to one gallon, then take out these barks, add to this two quarts of the best old rye whisky you can get. This is the greatest preventative of diseases we have ever known; the liquor is only to preserve this decoction; these bitters purify the blood, and give regular tone to the stomach. All persons may in safety use these bitters; dose, a half a wine glass full in the morning, at eleven o'clock, and the same at night.

MATERIA MEDICA.

SWEET FENNEL, THE ROOTS AND SEEDS.

This is a biennial plant, of which there are two varieties. The sweet fennel grows wild in Italy, but is cultivated in gardens in England. It is smaller in all its parts, than the common, except the seeds, which are considerable larger. The seeds of the two sorts differ, likewise, in shape and color. Those of the common are roundish, oblong, flattish on one side, and protuberant on the other, of a dark, almost blackish color. Those of the sweet are longer, narrower, not so flat, generally crooked, and of a whitish or pale yellowish color. The seeds of both the fennels have an aromatic smell, and a moderately warm, pungent taste, and also have a considerable degree of sweetness. The roots made into a tea is excellent in cases of colds, coughs, diarrhœa, &c. The oil of the seeds is a very excellent stimulous, and should be used in intermittent fevers, rheumatisms, gout, and any disease of the

lungs whatever; it should be taken in a little weak toddy. The oil applied externally, is good in cases of
white swelling, scrofula, and cancers.

ANGELICA, THE ROOTS AND SEEDS.

Angelica is a large, biennial, umbelliferous plant. It
grows spontaneously on the banks of rivers in Alpine
countries; but for the use of the shops, it is cultivated
in different parts of Europe. All the parts of angelica,
especially the roots, have a fragrant, aromatic smell, a
pleasant, bitterish, warm taste, glowing upon the lips
and palate for a long time after they have been chewed. The flavor of the seeds and leaves is very perish-
able, particularly that of the latter, which, on being
barely dried, lose the greater part of their taste and
smell; the roots are more tenacious of their flavor —
though they lose part of it with keeping. The fresh
roots, wounded early in the spring, yields an odorous,
yellow juice, which slowly exsiccated, proves an ele-
gant gummy resin, very rich in the virtues of the angelica. On drying the root, this juice concerts into
distinct moleculae, which, on cutting it longitudinally,
appear distributed in little veins; in this state they are
extracted by alchohol, but not by watery liquors. Angelica roots are apt to grow mouldy, and to be preyed
on by insects, unless thoroughly dried, kept in a dry
place, and frequently aired. Take a peck of the roots
of angelica, boil in two gallons of weak vinegar or
strong cider, to one quart; to this should be added one
pint of honey; this is a first rate preparation for pulmonary consumption. A strong tea made of the seeds is
excellent in cases of flooding, and will relieve pains in
the stomach and bowels. The oil made into a tincture
is one of the most foremost things in the Materia Medica, in cases of the gravel or any eruptions in the uterine vessels. ' An adult may take from a half to a tea

spoonful three times a day, in a little water. It may also be used in case of fits, or any spasmodic affections whatever. The leaves dried and pulverized, and made into pills, with a little sugar and water, is a good tonic for the stomach; two or three should be taken every day — it will also strengthen the nerves.

COMMON CAMOMILE, THE FLOWERS.

Camomile is a biennial plant, indigenous to the south of England, but is cultivated in many of our gardens. The flowers have a strong, not ungrateful, aromatic smell, and a very bitter, nausea taste. These are so very generally employed in medicine, as to render their extensive cultivation in the United States, well worthy of mankind. The single variety is best. Their active constituents are bitter, extractive and essential oil. To the latter is to be ascribed their anti-spasmodic, carminative, cordial, and diaphoretic effects; to the former their influence in promoting digestion. Medical use — Camomile flowers are a very common and excellent remedy, which is often used with advantage in spasmodic diseases, in hysteria, in spasmodic and flatulent colics, in suppression of the menstrual discharge, in the vomiting of puerperal women, and in the after pains; in gout, in podagra, in the intermittents, and in typhus. As camomile excites the peristatic motion, it is useful in dysentery, but it is not admissible in all cases of diarrhœa.

From its stimulating and somewhat unpleasant essential oil, camomile is also capable of exciting vomiting, especially when given in warm infusions; and in this way it is often used to assist the action of other emetics.

A cold infusion, made by suffering cold water to stand over the flowers for eight or ten hours before use, forms a most delightful drink, being divested of that

oil, which is very ungrateful to many in the warm infusion.

Externally, camomile flowers may be prepared in an
ointment, with hog's lard or sweet oil; is good to remove pains from the joints, should be rubbed on the
parts affected, warm by the fire every night and morning. An infusion of the flowers in the form of a tea,
drank warm, is excellent to promote the wenses,
wherein there is obstructions taken from cold. The
essential oil may be obtained by distillation; this possesses the anti-spasmodic powers in a high degree; by
making the oil in a tincture, it is an excellent medicine
in cases of weakness in the back, particularly with females. From ten to thirty drops may be taken three
times a day, it will also strengthen the whole digestive
powers of the system.

SOUTHERN WOOD.

This is a perennial shrub which grows readily in our
gardens though a native of the south of Europe. Southern wood has a strong smell, which to most of people is
not disagreeable, it has a pungent bitter and somewhat
nauseous taste. These qualities are very completely
extracted by alcohol, from the leaves and roots, and
the tincture is of a beautiful green color, this is
an excellect medicine, and should be freely used in all
cases of gonorrhea, flour albus, hemorrhage or flooding,
from ten to a hundred drops a day in a little water, may
be used, the quantity should be decreased or increased
as the nature of the case may require. The leaves
and roots make an excellent salve when combined with
dog's or buzzard's oil, it is good to heal all kinds of
ulcers, fresh cuts, burns, &c.

COMMON WORM WOOD.

This biennial herb grows by the road sides, and on

rubbish in many parts of Britain and about London, is cultivated for medical use, it is also a common shrub in many of our gardens, its smell is strong and disagreeable, its taste is intensely bitter, its active constituents are bitter excrative and essential oil, it is excellent in all complaints of the stomach, intermittent fevers, in cachexy, Hydrophic, Jaundice, Worms, &c. As the medical properties are most confined to the oil, it should be distilled. The oil is of a dark green color, and contains the whole flavor of the plant. In some cases it should be made into a tincture with alcohol, this should be given in cases of the Jaundice, fevers, &c., the tincture should be used in this form, the patient may take from ten to thirty drops, three or four times a day, in a little water. It is also excellent in cases of dyspepsia, cramp colics, in those cases it should be used as above mentioned, the oil is also good to destroy worms in children, from three to five drops should be given on a little sugar every night, for three or four nights in succession, I never have knew it to fail of having a good effect. I have relieved children with this simple oil when given out to die.

INDIAN TURNIP, ALSO CALLED DRAGGON ROOT.

As this herb is so well known through the western country by the citizens, it is not necessary to give a description of the plant, but only of its medical properties. The acrimony of the root of this plant, is well known. By the root being dried and pulverised, four ounces to one pint of honey or molasses, is good in cases of Asthma, Croup, Hoopingcough, Measles, &c., an adult in those cases may take half a table spoonful three times a day, children under ten years old, one tea spoonful.

The roots boiled in sweet milk is excellent for pains in the bowels, and particularly when there is difficulty

of making water. The roots and top stewed in hogs-
lard makes a good ointment, and may be advantageously used in cases of scald head, Ring or Teter worms.
It may also be used on the glands of the neck when
caused by cold, mumps or any general inflammation
whatever.

WILD GINGER, THE ROOT.

From the agreeable aromatic taste of the root, the
name of wild ginger has been given it. It is also called in some parts of the country, colt's-foot, the root by
distillation will yield a very bitter pungent volatile oil,
of a reddish color. This oil is a very great stimulons
and is good in weak debilitated cases of the stomach.
The oil by being used will increase the appetite and
produce digestion, dispel wind from the stomach, and
bowels, it should be taken from five to twenty drops a
day on a little loaf sugar. The roots made into a strong
tea, will break the intermittent fever, it should be
drank freely every night at bed time until it relieves the
complaint.

BUTTERFLY WEED, PLEURISY ROOT.

This is one of the most beautiful perennial plants,
flourishing best in a light sandy soil, by the way side,
under fences, and near old stumps in rye fields, there
are sometimes fifteen or twenty or more stalks the size
of a pipe stem, proceeding from one root, rising from
one to two feet in height, and spreading to a considerable extent, generally in a recumbent position, the stalks
are round and wooly, of a reddish brown color on the
sun side, the leaves stand irregularly and are spear or
tongue shaped, with a short foot stalk, and covered
with a fine down on the under surface, the umbels are
compact at the extremities of the branches, and formed like the common silk weed, but differing from it in

the color of the flowers, being of a beautiful bright orange color, while those of the silk weed are of a pale purplish hue, the flowers appear in July and August and are distinguished by their size and brilliancy from all the flowers of the field, these are succeeded by long and slender pods containing the seeds, which have a delicate kind of silk attached to them, this is propably the only variety of asclepias that is destitute of a milky juice, the root is spindle or carrot shape, of a light brownish color on the outer surface, white coarse and streaked within.

This herb makes one of the best medicines that I have ever used in cases of the pleurisy. The root should be boiled in water to a strong liquid or tea, and may be taken from a table spoonful to a wine glass full three times a day. I have relieved cases of pleurisy with this medicine, when every thing else failed, and the patient given out to die. The root pulverized, is a very mild excellent purgative, given in doses from ten to fifteen grains to an adult. The roots beat fine and applied to the back of the neck, will ease pain in the head, shoulders, or arms. And when it is rubbed all over the system, it will produce a general warmth which is very necessary in many cases. When taken as a tea, is excellent in cases of cholera-morbus. An extract of it, in a tincture of French brandy or Alcohol is excellent in cases of chronic rheumatism, and should be taken from a tea, to a half a table spoonful two or three times a day.

COMMON SILK WEED, THE ROOT.

From the abundance of its milky juice this has also been called milk weed, the leaves are spear or tongue shaped and the blossoms are of a reddish purple color and they are exhibited at the extremeties of the branches, the seeds are contained in oblong pods, and are crowded with down extremely fine and soft, resembling silk which has occasioned the name of silk weed, the stalk of this species, is from three to six feet high, the leaves are large, standing on large foot stalks, a milky juice exudes from the stem or leaves when broken the root as soon as it penetrates the earth, shoots off horrizontally and often sends out other stalks; it abounds round fences and road sides in many parts of our country.

It has a bitter aromatic taste. This is a very excellent and powerful tonic. And may be advantageously used in Typhus, nervous and dropsical cases. The root should be pulverized when used in the above cases, and may be taken in doses, from two to four grains, four or five times a day. It will break the fevers, and cleanse the stomach, purge the blood, strengthen the nerves, operates mildly on the bowels, produces action on the gall, and keeps a regular circulation on the liver. When this root is reduced to powder and taken in doses from half to a tea spoonful is very good in cases of a snake or spider bite—each dose may be mixed with a little honey. It may also be advantageously used in cases of dropsy and piles—and a small handful of this root put to a quart of good spirits may prove quite beneficial in the breast complaint. I know a Doctor who was cured of a pain in his breast by using this root one week—He says that the way he prepared it, was by boiling a hand ful of it in water down to three gills, and added half a pint of honey to the liquor, and simmered it a minute or two over a slow fire, and then bottled it, and used a table spoonful three times a day, living at the same time on light diet.

N. B. Previous to the adding of the honey, the liquor must be strained through a flannel cloth.

AMERICAN CENTAURY.

It is a beautiful annual plant abundant in many parts

of the United States, every part of it is a pure an^d strong bitter which properly is communicated alike t^o alcohol and water. It is a very powerful astringent, it is a useful tonic and a promoter of digestion, and may be emyloyed successfully in case of yellow, intermitent and remittent fever. It is a remedy the Indians apply greatly to, in cases of diarrhœa. The extract of the root with alcohol should be freely used in all cases of fever.

WORM SEED, JERUSALEM OAK,

This plant grows plentifuly in the United States and is much used for worms. The whole plant has a powerful smell of which it is very retentive, its taste bitter, with much aromatic acrimony. The whole plant may be employed, the express juice is used in doses of a table spoonful for a child two or three years old. A decoction of the plant, made by boiling a handful of the green leaves in a quart of milk for about one quarter of an hour to which orange peels may be added and given to a child four or five years old, in doses about a wine glass full two or three times a day. The seeds may also be employed, reduced to a fine powder and made into an electuary, with syrup, of this a child of two or three years old may take a table spoonful early in the morning, abstaining from nourishment for some hours, a light dose may be given at night, it is often necessary to continue this course for several days.— The essential oil made of the seeds are equally efficacious, and should be taken from three to five drops on a little sugar once or twice a day. This is a great medicine to destroy the worms, and should be kept by all persons who have families, and freely used when necessary.

HORSE RADISH, THE ROOT.

This perennial plant is sometimes found wild about river sides and other moist places, is also cultivated in our gardens. It flowers in June. Horse radish root has a quick pungent smell and a penetrating acrid taste. It nevertheless contains in certain vessels, a sweet juice which sometimes exudes upon the surface. By drying, it loses all its acrimony, becomes at first sweetish and afterwards almost insipid. If kept in a cool place covered with sand it retaines its qualities for considerable time. This root is an extreme penetrating stimulous, it excites the solids and promotes the fluid secretions. It may be advantageously used in cases of scurvy, likewise in dropsies, in particular those which follow intermittent fevers. The medical properties of the root should be extracted by alcohol, this may be done by beating the root and adding the spirit to it, keeping the same cosely stopped in a bottle for two or three days, it is then fit for use, and may be freely used as the nature of the case may require. The root pulverized and formed into snuff will stop bleeding at the nose, and ease pains in the head, it is also good to cut off film from the eyes, the root roasted in the fire and then beat fine while warm, and drank in French brandy will produce deliverance of a child, when many other remedies may fail. The leaves bound to risings, sprains, burns, cuts. &c., wet in a little vinegar may be advantageously used.

COMMON SCURVY GRASS, TONGUE GRASS.

This annual plant which grows at the sides of cliffs round fences in meadows. is also cultivated in gardens, when it is fresh it has a peculiar smell especially when bruised and a kind of saline acrid taste, which it loses completely by drying, but which it imparts by distilla-

tion, it yields an essential oil, the smell of which is ex_
tremely pungent the fresh plant is a gentle stimulent and
diuretic. It may be employed externally, as a garglin
sore throat and scorbutic affections of the gums. When
formed into a solution, it is excellent to be used in cases
of salivation, where the tongue and mouth are very sore.
The oil is excellent in cases of the gravel, and auy debility of the kidneys whatever, it will greatly increase
the urine. It should be taken from five to twenty
drops, two or three times a day, in any of those cases,
it should be taken in a strong tea made of parsnips or
tongue grass.

COMMON HEMLOCK OR GARDEN HEMLOCK.

This is a large biennial umbelliferous plant which
grows commonly about the sides of fields, under hedges and moist shady places, the stalk is often three, four
and even six feet high, hollow, smooth not beset with
hairs and marked with red or brown spots, the leaves
are large and have long and thick foot stalks which at
the lower end assumes the form of a groove, surround
the stem from each side of the foot stalk, other foot
stalks arise, and from these a still smaller order on
which there are dark green shining, lancet shaped,
notched leaves.

The flowers consists of five white heart shaped leaves
The seeds are flat on the one side and hemispherical on
the other. Hemlock's should not be gathered unless
its peculiar smell be strong, the leaves should be collected in the month of June when the plant is in its
flower. The leaves are then to be dried quick in a hot
sun or rather on tin plates before the fire, and preserved in bags or strong brown paper. Fresh hemlock
contains not only the narcotic, but also the acrid prin-
cipals of the latter, the whole plant is somewhat poisonous when taken in over doses, it produces vertigo,
dimness of sight, difficulty of speech, nauseous vomit-

ing, anxiety, spasms, &c. Though it may be used with
propriety and safety and with great success. The
leaves when dried and pulverized and formed into pills
is an active purgative and may be, used with safety.
The root when distilled yields an essential oil, the stalk,
leaves, &c., may be distilled with the roots, this oil applied externally will cure the tetter or ring worm and
also the scald head, but it should be weakened with
spirits, it is also excellent in cases of rheumatism, it
should be rubbed on the joints every night and morning. This oil in cases of rheumatisms when applied as
directed, have almost performed miracles. I relieved
a man who came to me from Lexington, the distance
of fifty miles, he was nine days coming, sometimes on
his knees then his crutches, and through great difficulty
he arrived at my house, he had been afflicted with the
chronic rheumatism for about two years, which had
disabled him from doing any kind of business whatever.
The joints were all completely swelled and his person
much drawn and disfigured. He stayed in my neighborhood three weeks during which time I attended on
him. I used this oil all over him externally from the
sole of the foot to the crown of the head every night
and morning at the same time giving him a tincture of
gum guiacum and mild purgatives, this course of treatment entirely relieved him to the astonishment of all
the neighborhood and those who seen him, he walked
back to Lexington in a day and a half. Tho' this poor
man had not a dollar in the world and was looked upon
as a vagabond owing to his affliction. Since he got well
he is accumulating more property than any citizen in
the city of Lexington. I have relieved many of this
awful disease by pursuing the same course. The oil
when formed into a tincture is one of the best medicines in all the materia medica for the obstruction of
the menses produced by cold. It should be taken from
ten to thirty drops three times a day. The abdomen
should be bathed in an ointment made of camomile

flowers every night. By pursuing this course it will produce that regular discharge that nature requires. It is also excellent in cases of hysterics.

DOG WOOD, THE BARK.

This beautiful shrub is found in every part of the United States. In the New England States it is known by the name of box-wood. The bark is a very considerable astringent, and should be used in all cases of diarrhœa and intermittent fevers. The Indians employ it in all kinds of fevers with a great deal of success. The berries distilled, yield a dark brownish colored oil, which is excellent in cases of chronic diseases of the liver, dyspepsia, and indigestion of the stomach; from ten to twenty drops of the oil should be used three times a day, in a little water. A decoction of the leaves or blossoms, made strong, is good in cases of flooding.

SWAMP, OR SKUNK CABBAGE, THE ROOT.

Not many persons who are acquainted with the skunk cabbage — the multitude of large, rank growing leaves from one single root. It grows in swamps, meadows, and near fences and lanes, &c., and may be bought at the botanical shops. The sensible properties of this herb, gives it a place in this materia medica — every part of the plant is a powerful anti-spasmodic. The root pulverized, made into a powder, is excellent in cases of asthma, pulmonist, scrofula, and diabetes; from five to ten grains may be taken three times a day, in a little honey. The bruised leaves are excellent applied to ulcers, wounds, and all cutaneous disorders, such as ulcerations. The juice applied to herpes is an immediate cure. The leaves are also good to dress

12

blisters, &c. The leaves made into a tea is good in cases of hysterics, hypochondriac, pains in the stomach and intestines.

PAILADELPHIA FLEA-BANE, THE PLANT.

This is one of the most common plants in our country — it grows in fields and meadows; The plant is two or three feet in height, much branched at the top. The root is branched, somewhat fibrous, and of a yellowish cast; the upper leaves and flowers are numerous, of a whitish and rather a blue color. It begins to flower in July and continues till August. The leaves, flowers, and roots, act as a powerful sudorific and diuretic. It may be advantageously used in cases of dropsy; a strong tea made of the roots, leaves and flowers, will carry off waters in case of dropsies, when used in a strong tea. The flowers alone are excellent, to be used in a decoction of French brandy — for the gout or king's evil. The roots pulverized into a powder are good in cases of burning in the stomach, colics and jaundice, and should be taken from a tea to a table spoonful three times a day. It will also act mildly on the bowels as a purgative.

THOROUGHWORT, BONESET, INDIANSAGE.

This plant is known by the name of through-stem, bross-wort, Indian sage, and is used a great deal among the Indians in cases of fever as an emetic. This is a native annual plant, flourishing abundantly in wet meadows and other moist places. The stalk is hairy, and rises from two to four feet in height, the flowers are white and appear in July and August, forming a corymbus at the termination of the branches, the leaves at each joint are horizontal from three to four inches long, and about an inch broad, at the base gradually lessening to a very acute point of a dark green and covered with short hairs. Thoroughwort certainly possesses active properties as an emetic, sudorific, sometimes as a purgative. The root pulverised and taken in a little molasses or honey is good in case of phthisic, croup, &c., should be used according as the case may require. A water infusion of the leaves made warm is a very excellent emetic, and should be freely used in every case of the stomach where there appears to be too great a collection of improper bile. The flowers also form excellect ointment combined with hog's lard or buzzard's oil, this is excellent to heal all kinds of ulcers, sores, sore throats, &c. &c.

COMMON OR WILD HOREHOUND.

This plant grows in abundance in many parts of our country. As it is so well known to the citizens of the country it is not necessary to give any description of the herb, only its medical qualities, it is one of the great tonics of our western country, and should be freely used in all cases where fevers are broke, to nourish and strengthen the system. The leaves should be beat fine and mixed with wine, and should be freely used in all weak and debilitated cases. The root pulzerised and mixed with honey is good to break a cold and to produce an expectoration from the lungs, and at the same time will strengthen the stomach, &c.

MOUNTAIN TEA OR PARTRIDGE BERRY.

It is also called berry tea and by some deer berries. It is extensively spread over the more barren mountaneous parts of the United States. As it is so well known by the people generally, it is not necessary to say but little respecting its description. The root, leaves, and berries distilled yields an essential oil, which may be advantageously used in cases of coughs, colds, consumptions, obstructions of the system in general. From five to fifteen drops of the oil should be taken on a little loaf sugar two or three times a day. The leaves boiled to a strong tea are excellent to be used in cases of flour albus or whites. The berries when completely boiled and thickened with honey and flour, equal quantities, forms an excellent salve for cancers, sore legs, stone bruises, ulcers from scrofula, and any risings whatever.

INDIAN PHYSIC.

This shrub grows plentifully in the United States and is one of the few active plants of the class Scosandria. the root, which is generally employed, is equal or superior to the ipecacuanha, the active powers seem to reside excessively in the root, it is a safe efficacious emetic, in doses of about thirty grains, it also possesses a tonic power and may be used very beneficially in intermittent fevers, it is sometimes very injudiciously employed by the ccuntry, people in so much they are obliged to apply for medical aid, to remove the debility produced by over portions of the root. It should be taken in small portions until it vomits freely, when used in this way there is no danger to be apprehended. It not only removes the overportion of bile from the stomach, but strengthens the digestive powers of the system. When it is used in small broken doses it is good for pains in the stomach, side, back and head, and will also produce a free expectoration from the lungs when it is produced from cold.

YELLOW ROOT.

This is a common plant in various parts of the United States, the root is a very powerful bitter, and when dried it has a strong virose smell, a spirituous infusion of the root is a very excellent tonic and should be freely used in all cases of scrofula. It cleanses the stomach, purifies the blood and acts upon the uterine vessels. The roots pulverised into a powder is greatly among the Indians in all cases of cancers and indeed very successfully too. I have tried the effects of this powder myself in cases of cancers, and at all times with great success. The leaves boiled in strong vinegar say two pounds of the leaves in half a gallon of vinegar boiled to half a pint is excellent in cases of snake bites, particularly where there is any inflammation arisen, from half to a table spoonful should be taken thrice a day. It may be increased or decreased as the nature of the case may require. The juice of the leaves when beat is good for fits, a wine glass full should be drank two or three times a day, this has relieved many when given up to die.

PUCCOON ROOT, OR BLOOD ROOT.

The puccoon root may be very easily known as it has a peculiar reddish or rather an orange colored juice which pervades every part of it, it is one of the most beautiful and delicate vegetables of our country, it is particularly interesting from its flowering at a season when there is little or no general verdure, and scarcely anything in bloom except trees, which renders this plant very attractive. It is also one of the most abundant plants in our State and generally grows in rich bottom land. and on the sides of hills creeks and branches. This plant is an emetic and a purgative, though it should be cautiously used, yet it may be used with impunity either as an emetic or purgative. The root should be boiled to a strong decoction in the form of tea, it is excellent to be taken in this way, particularly in cases of cramp colic, bilious colic, cholera morbus or an inflammation in the bowels, from a table spoonful to a wine

glass full should be drank warm in any of those cases.
The juice extracted is good to put in weak eyes to
strengthen them, is also good for the tooth ache, and
for sore mouth.   The juice when mixed with a little
laudanum or sweet oil is a sure remedy for a pain in
the ear.

COMMON HEN-BANE.

Hen-bane is an annual plant which grows in great
abundance in many parts of our western country, it
genearally grows by the road sides and among rubbish,
it flowers in July, its smell is strong and peculiar, and
when bruised someting like tobacco especially when
the leaves are burnt, and on burning they sparkle as if
they contained a nitrat, when chewed however they
have no saline taste, but are insipid mild and pleasant.
Hen-bane is a narcotic and sudorific, and may be freely
used in any case where it is necesary,
The root when pulverized and formed into a decoction with wine is one of the most powerful medicines to
act upon the nervous system that I have ever tried, it
will cure the nervous fever, and any debility of the
nerves whatever.   It is great in case of nervous colic
or wind in the blood, it produce a sweets perspiration
through the whole system at the same time acts gently
upon the bowels.   It will also produce a flow of urine,
and strengthen the stomach.   It is also good for the
jaundice or an obstruction of the gall.   It may also be
used in cases of the consumption, (of the liquid as described) it should be taken from a table spoonful to a
wine glassful two or three times a day.   If in case it
should act too powerful on the system a less quantity
may be taken.   The Indians use this preparation in all
nervous affections whatever, and generally with a great
deal of success.   The leaves bruised and applied to any
iflammation or swelling, externally, is also useful.

COMMON HYSOP.

Hysop is a perenial herb which grows wild in Germany, though it is cultivated in our gardens in America. Its leaves have an aromatic smell and a warm pungent taste. The virtues depend entirely on the essential oil which rises by distillation. This oil is excellent in cases of bleeding of the lungs, it should be mixed in a little sugar, and should be taken from ten to twenty drops three or four times a day. It is good in case of hoarseness and colds. This oil when combined with pulverized cinnamon is excellent in cases of flooding. It should be made in a tincture, take one fourth of an ounce of the oil, one ounce of cinnamon, three ounces of alcohol, this should be shook well together, it is then fit for use, the dose should be from a tea to half a table spoonful, it may be increased or decreased as the nature of the case may be.

ELECAMPANE ROOT.

This is a very large, downy, perenial plant, sometimes found wild in moist, rich soils — it flowers in July and August; this plant is known to most of persons, therefore a description is unnecessary. The root has an agreeable, aromatic smell — its taste on first chewing is gluttonous, and, as it were, somewhat ranked. In a little time it discovers an aromatic bitterness, considerbly acrid. This root is excellent in case of consumption, icterious disorders, also in cases of scrofula. It should be boiled till the strength is entirely extracted from the root, the liquid should then be strained, and to every quart should be added a gill of honey, one grain of rifined nitre, or salt petre, one ounce of Holland gin ; this is good in all weak and debilitated cases of the system whatever; one table spoonful should be taken three times per day, living at the same time on light diet. The roots, when made into a strong tea equally combined with sarsaparilly and sassafras, drank at night, is a great remedy for venerial diseases.

AMERICAN JUNIPER

This is an ever green shrub, growing on healthy and hilly grounds, in many parts of our country ; the berries have a strong, but not disagreeable smell, and a warm pungent sweet taste, which if they are long chewed, or previously bruised, is followed by a bitterish taste. It is seldom more than two or three feet high, the root, leaves, and berries, yield oil by distillation, which is very stimulating carminatives. An infusion of the leaves, is a great remedy in cases of dropsy of the abdomen, it operates merely on the bowels, and upon the uterine vessels, I have relieved many cases of dropsy by only giving this simple remedy. The oil should be made into a tincture when used, and should be freely used in all cases of dropsy, from thirty to fifty drops of this tincture should be taken three or four times a day, living at the same time on light diet. The oil is good in cases of white swelling, it should be rubbed all over the affected parts, every night and morning; this oil alone has cured many cases of white swelling. being applied in this way, and at the same time living on light diet, and taking light purgatives ; it will do well to try this medicine before the patient has his leg or thigh taken off.

LOBELIA INFLATIA, INDIAN TOBACCO, THE HERB.

The Lobelia inflatia is indigenous and annual, rising from one to two feet in height, with branched stems. The leaves are oblong, alternate : slightly serrated and sessile. The blossoms are solitary, in a kind of spike, of a pale blue color. It is found common in dry fields, among barley and rye stubble, and flowers in July and August; its pods are small, and filled with numerous small seeds. The leaves chewed are at first insipid, but soon becomes pungent, occasioning a copious discharge of saliva. If they are held in the mouth for some time, they produce a slight giddiness and pain in the head, with a trembling agitation of the whole body ; at length (if a small portion of the chewed leaves be swallowed,) they bring on extreme nausea and vomiting. This plant is possessed of very active qualities, notwithstanding the violent effects from chewing the leaves, and may be used to great advantage in many cases ; and may be ranked as one among the foremost plants in the materia medica, and forms a valuable medicine in the cure of asthma, and other complaints of the human system. This plant was employed by the aborigines as an emetic, and its properties have very frequently been subjected to the test of practical experiment. It is found to operate as a speedy and active emetic, and it often induces a most profuse perspiration, immediately after being received into the stomach. It has proved serviceable in cases of colic, where emetics were indicated. It is probably one of the most powerful vegetable substances with which we are acquainted, and no rational practitioner will have recourse to it, but with the greatest precaution, although when properly and cautiously administered, proves both beneficial and efficacious in the removal of diseases. The dose usually prescribed for an adult is from five to ten grains, of the powdered leaves and pods, and the quantity necessary for a child must be regulated according to their age, from three to five grains may be given to a child of six years of age. The most proper form of administering the emetic powder, is to take a sufficiency for a dose and put it in a bowl and add about a half a pint of water, blood warm. and make three drinks of this at intervals of ten minutes, and the same repeated till the desired operation is produced.

13

' SASSAFRAS BARK, THE ROOT, ESSENTIAL OIL.

This tree is a native of America, it is of a soft light and spongy texture, of a rusty white color, of a strong pleasant smell, and a sweetish aromatic taste. The trees in places grow to a considerable height, but we frequently find small shrubs of the same kind on the side of hills, in thickets, and poor ground; it is from three to five feet high, the leaves of a pleasant taste, the outside bark of the root, of a dark, rough appearance. Sassafras, from its quantity of volatile oil, contains gentle stimulating, heating, sudorific and diuretic properties. The essential oil may be obtained by distillation, it is of a whitish yellow color, and sinks in water. It is highly stimulating and heating, and must be given only in very small doses. It is very useful in cases of intermittent fevers ; take half an ounce of the oil, forty grains of quinine, half an ounce of alcohol, shake it together, and take from half a tea spoonful to a tea spoonful two or three times a day in a little weak tody, it will break any kind of chills or agues in the course of two or three days, though it should be pursued until the complaint is entirely removed. The essential oil is a great remedy in case of wens, it should be rubbed on warm by the fire every night and morning, it has cured many of that unpleasant disease.

COW PARSNIP, OR MASTER WORT

This is a perennial plant of our country, it grows in hedges near fences, the stalk is a large, tubular, invested with a down which also covers the leaves, which are large and jagged, five on each stalk, and very much the color of worm wood; it flowers in June, the roots are divided into several long and fibrous branches, resembling a large parsley root, and the height of the plant in its maturity may he from two to four feet high. The root has a rank strong smell, and pungent taste. The particular complaint in which this herb is good, is in epileptic fits; it is one of the most foremost things in the garden of nature, for that malancholy and sad complaint. The root should be pulverized, and from three to five grains may be taken two or three times a day in a little strong pennyroal tea, while taking this medicine, there should be half a pint of blood taken out of the arm every day, this course should be pursued eight or ten days. I have never known it to fail in performing a cure; the patient should be cautious in taking cold, no diet should be used, only gruel and soup. The leaves boiled to a strong decoction and made into a salve with tallow, and turpentine equal quantities, is a great salve in cases of burns; it will extract the fire from the system in a few minutes, and ease the pains at the same time, it should be kept by all families for that purpose.

TULIP TREE, OR POPLAR

It is a native and well known tree in the U. States, called also American poplar, it attains to a very large size, rising as high as any tree of the forest, and makes a noble and beautiful appearance when in flower about the middle of May; this tree is remarkable for the shape of its leaves, having the middle lobe of the three truncate, or cut transversely at the end; the flowers are large and bell shaped, of three leaves, six petals to the crolla, marked with green yellow and red spots, and many lance shaped seeds lying one over another and forming a sort of cone. The bark of the root is a great tonic, and should be used in all weak and debilitated cases of the system. The inside bark of the root should be finely pulverized—and should be taken from three to ten grains once or twice a day, when used freely it operates mildly on the bowels. The root boiled to a strong liquid, strained, and a quart of honey added to the gallon, is an excellent remedy in cases of dropsy of the breast, and should be taken from a table spoonful to a wine glass full three times a day.   The bark yields an essential oil by distillation, of a whitish dark color it has a beautiful perfume and pleasant to the ta.te, and is good in cases of dyspepsia, and disorders of the liver, weakness of the back, it should be taken from five to twenty drops two or three times a day in a little syrup, the oil applied externally is good to strengthen the joints.   A tea made of the blossoms is excellent for Hysterical affections.

PEPPERMINT.

This species of mint is perennial and also a native of our country, it is cultivated in great quantities in Britain for the essential oil, the leaves have a strong, rather agreeable smell, and intensely pungent aromatic taste, resembling that of pepper and accompanied with a peculiar sensation of coldness.   The oil is a very considerable stimulus and should be freely used in cases of cramp colic, and dysentery.   A strong tea made of the leaves is good to stop vomiting or water brash.

VIRGINIA BROOM RAPE, OR BEECH DROPS.

This plant is common in many parts of the United States, it generally grows among beech timber and in shady ground, it is from three to nine inches high, two or three little stems puts off from the herb two or three inches from the ground, has several small leaves on each branch, though these leaves in a short time drop off, and the shrub is left naked, it is extremely bitter to the taste, it is a great astringent, and should be freely used in cases of dysentery, or flooding, it should be boiled in new sweet milk to a strong tea, and should be taken from a wine glassful to a gill, two or three times a day. The root boiled in beer or wine is excellent in diseases of the kidneys, particularly where there is a pain on each side where the kidneys lay, a table spoon. ful should be taken every night and moring. The root pulverized into a powder, is good to put into a cancer to eat out the root and heal up the ulcer, and may be advantageously used in eating out the proud flesh of any sores.

WOOD SORREL, THE LEAVES.

This is a small perennial plant which grows wild in the woods and shady hedges, the leaves contain a con- siderable quantity of acid and have an extremely pleas- ant taste, they possess the power of vegetable acids in general. This little herb boiled in weak vinegar to a strong liquid, to which there should be added a small portion of the rust of iron, this should be given to all young females, about the time of menstruation; this will prevent any difficulty from taking place, and in all probability will secure the young lady's health through life. It should be taken for three or four months in succession, until they become entirely regular; by pur- suing this course the lives of many young ladies may be preserved, one table spoonful may be taken three times a day just before meal time. The diet should be light, and the feet frequently bathed in warm water. The juice of the leaves is good in cases of weakness of the stomach, and also should be applied externally in cases of the bites of Dogs, or any other venimous animal.

POKE, THE LEAVES, BERRIES AND ROOTS.

This is one of the most common plants in all our country, and well known by the citizens in general, it has a thick fleshy perennial root, as large as parsnips, from this rise many purplish stalks about an inch thick and six or seven feet long, which breaks into many branches, irregular set, with large oval sharp pointed leaves supported on short foot stalks, these are at first of a fresh green color, but as they grow old they turn reddish, these are succeeded by round depressed berries, having ten cells each of which contains a single smooth seed. A tincture of the ripe berries in brandy or wine is a great remedy is cases of sciatic, or chronic rheumatisms, and should be freely used in all such cases. The leaves boiled to a strong tea, with the addition of a small portion of the tincture of gum guiacum is good in cases of the small pox, a gill should be drank three times a day, this preparation has cured many of that complaint. The juice of the berries is a mild purgative and is good in all cases of costiveness of the bowels; The juice should be simmered down by the fire until it becomes nearly as thick as honey, from a half to a table spoonful should be taken as the nature of the case may require.

The green root beat fine is excellent to be applied to the feet, ancles, or any other part of the system, it is almost equal to spanish flies. Though it does not produce the same effect on the skin. An extraction of the root with French brandy is a good emetic and may be used with entire safety, while it is operating the patient should drink freely of gruel or warm water. The root boiled to a strong decoction and thickened with flour, honey, eggs and sweet oil, forms a great salve for the white swelling or any running ulcer or sore.

GREEN PLANTAIN, THE LEAVES.

This herb is very common through all our country, it grows in yards, by the side of fences, in hedges sunshiny places, &c. It flowers from June to August the leaves are good to be applied to bruises, slight wounds, inflamed sore eyes. The juice is good for poisons: I knew a man who was bit by a rattle snake, in ten minutes afterwards was completely blind and almost speechless, a gill of the juice of the leaves were poured down his throat and in twenty minutes he was able to speak distinctly, in twenty minutes more the same quantity was administered which gave great relief indeed. There was some of the leaves applied to the place externally — in three hours from that time, at the same time he took a gill of the juice in the same quantity of new warm sweet milk, and in the course of a few days was entirely well, and another case of a gentleman, who was bitten about the knee by a venimous spider, in a few minutes he observed a pain shooting upward from the spot, which immediately appeared to reach his heart, a quantity of plantain leaf was immediately procured and the juice being bruised out was swallowed largely by which the progress of the poison soon was arrested, and a final cure effected. A strong tea made of the leaves is good in cases of the croup hoopingcough, measles, &c.

MAY-APPLE, OR MANDRAKE.

This plant is very common throughout all America, the fruit is excellent, and by many thought delicious. The leaves are rather of a poisonous nature. The root is an excellent purgative, in doses of twenty grains pulverized, the root boiled into a strong liquid equally combined with Philadelphia flea-bane, or white blossoms, this is a great medicine in cases of the dropsy, particu-

and a wine glass full to be taken two or three times a day, should it operate too severely on the bowels a less quantity should be taken, it may be increased or decreased as the case may require. The leaves dried and pulverized fine with the same quantity of rhubarb formed into pills makes a quick and mild purgative on the bowels, at the same time strengthen the stomach and producing expectoration from the lungs, in severe cases of cold.

SENECA SNAKE-ROOT OR RATTLF SNAKE-ROOT.

Senca is a perennial plant growing spontaneously in different parts of the western country, this root is usually about the size of the little finger, variously bent and contorted, and appears as if composed of joints, whence it is supposed to resemble the tail of the animal whose name it bears. A kind of membranous margin runs on each side the whole length of the root. It is an active stimulus, and increases the force of the circulation especially of the pulmonary vessls. A strong tea made of the root is good to be taken in cases of cold to produce perspiration and sweat. It is good to be taken in cases of female obstructions, particularly when caused by cold. The root pulverized to a fine powder and mixed with honey, is good in cases of Asthma or pulmonary consumption. Twenty grains of the root will act mildly on the bowels two or three times and will leave the bowels in a good situation.

GREAT BRISTORT OR SNAKE WEED.

This plant is perennial and grows in moist meadows, the root is about as thick as the little finger, of a blackish brown color on the outside and reddish within, the root is one or two inches thick and some cf them six inches long, it tapers off very small at the little end something like calamus. This root is a great astringent and should be used in all cases of flooding or spitting of blood, and Dysentery, venerial disease, the root should be boiled to a strong tea and may be taken, from a wine glassful to a gill two or three times a day, in any of those cases above mentioned. The juice of the leaves is good in cases of child bed fever, to allay the inflammation, a table spoonful of the juice should be taken every three hours until the fever and every inflammatoin subsides. I was called to see a woman not long since who had this fever, that was given out to die by six other Doctors, when I went she was completely swelled from her feet to her head, large purple spots on her face, head and arms, she was expected to die every minute. I immediately gave her one table spoonful of this juice combined with two grains of the sugar of lead, which gave her considerable ease in thirty minutes, I then repeated the same dose and at the same time wetting the leaves in vinegar, and binding them all over the abdomen, by pursuing this course of treatment for two days and nights the woman was entirely relieved.

WINTER BERRY.

This is a very common shrub in may parts of the United States, it grows in the greatest perfection in swamps, marshy, low grounds, side of branches particularly among grapevines, its leaf is something like a bramble brier leaf, its berries deep green through the winter, therefore it is called winter berry. The bark is manifestly an astringent, is likewise a considerable bitter, and pungent taste. The berry greatly partakes of the bitter quality and if infused in winen or brandy may be advantageously employed in cases where bitter tinctures are necessary, the bark may be used as a substitute for peruvian, in intermittent fevers, and in all other cases where barks should be given. A strong decoction of the root bolled, should be freely used in cases of gangreene or mortification, a wine glassful should be taken two or three times a day. At the same time keeping the bowels open with salts. This medicine will stop a mortification of the bowels (or intestines) quicker than any medicine I have ever used when taken inwardly. The same decoction should be applied externally on the parts affected. It should be combined with a small portion of sulphuric ether.— The root when distilled yields a darkish colored oil— resembling the oil of wormwood. This oil applied externally will kill all kinds of humors of the skin, and when it is made in a tincture is excellent in negro poison. Should be taken from ten to fifty drops two or three times a day, this has cured that disorder when all other means have failed.

PIPSISIWAY OR WINTER GREEN.

This herb grows on mountaneous land and on pine plains, when the box berry or cheek berry is found plenty it is an ever green shrub, and grows from three to six inches high, has a number of dark green leaves about half an inch wide, and from one to two inches long, with a scolloped edge, bears several seeds resembling allspice, the tops and roots possess medical properties, the roots when chewed are very pungent which will be felt for some time on the tongue afterwards, a strong tea made of this plant is good for cancers and all scrofulous humors, the root by distillation yields an oil which is very useful in cases of consumption or suppression of the menses, when used for the consumption it should be taken in a little syrup from ten to forty drops two or three times a day. When used for suppression the same quantity should be taken in strong ginger tea.

BUTTER NUT, WHITE WALNUT

This tree grows common in this country, and is well known from the nut which it bears, of an oblong shape,

and nerly as large as an egg, in which there is a meat
containing much oil, and is very good to the taste.—
The bark taken from the body of the tree or roots and
boiled down till thick may be made into pills, they op-
perate mildly on the bowels, a syrup made by boiling
the bark and adding one thiridmolasses and a little spirit
is good to give children in cases of worms. The buds
and twigs many also be used in the same case, that is
to destroy worms. The nuts diyed and the outside
bark taken off, then broke to pieces yield a quantity
of oil by distilation, which is superior to the castor oil
and may be taken in less quanties, it does not cramp
the bowels in the least, but works mild and pleasant
and may be used with entire safety.

BLACK-PERRY, THE BARK OF THE ROOT.

As this shrub is so extensively know it is not necessary to desciibe it. It is a very powerful astringent and
is good in cases of the pock where it has been running
on the system for some time, it should be used in the
form of a strong tea and the whole body should be
bathed in the same every night and morning, at the
same time keeping the bowels open with mild purgatives,
it is also good in cases of dropsy if it should check the
bowels too soon, a small dose of salts should be taken
and the same course pursued again, until a cure is performed. The bark of the root pulverized and made into pills is excellent in cases of the yellow Jaundice, two
of the pills should be taken every night.

RUE, THE HERP.

This is a small shrubby plant, a native of the south
of Europe and is cultivated in our gardens. Rue has a
strong and grateful smell, and a bitterish penetrating

taste, the leaves when in full vigor are extremely acrid insomuch as to inflame and blister the skin, if much handled. Rue by distillation yields a volatile oil which congeals readily, and may be obtained in great abundance. The oil possesses a stimulating and heating nature, and is serviceable in all spasmodic affections, and obstructed secretions ; the oil when formed and made into a tincture is good in cases of hysterics and fits. It should be used from ten to fifty drops, every night and morning in a little tar water. It is also good in cases where a woman is in travail and the pains are too slow. By giving a tea spoonful of this tincture every ten minutes will increase, the pain immediately and bring on deliverance.

I was called to see a case of this kind not long since where every thing had failed in producing deliverance and the woman given up to die, so soon as I got to the place I gave a tea spoonful of this tincture in a little weak toddy and in twenty minutes the little stanger was heard to halloo. This preparation may be used with safety,it will be well for mothers in that line to always have this preparation by them insomuch as its utility in female cases is wonderful and beyond description.

COMMON ELDER, THE FLOWERS, &c.

This shrub grows in hedges, along old fences, in pastures, meadows, &c. It flowers in May and ripens its fruit in September; the berries have a sweet taste, and are very pleasant. The juice of the berries is a quick and mild purgative. The juice, when simmered down slow to the consistency of mollasses, and a small portion of sugar added to it, is good in cases of consumption ; a tea spoonful should be taken three times a day, mixed with half a tea spoonful of fresh butter or sweet oil; this will strengthen the lungs, and heal the ulcers, and produce an expectoration of matter;

also, ease the cough, and will keep the bowels in a
proper state. The flowers made into a strog tea, and
drank freely, promotes the menses and removes ob.
structions. The bark of the root boiled very strong,
will remove swelling of the legs, by being bathed in it
warm, it also makes a good salve when mixed with lin.
seed oil, tallow, and opodeldoc, for any kind of a rising,
or cutaneous affections of any kind.

PRICKLY ASH, OR TOOTH ACHE TREE.

The bark is a very powerful stimulent, and exerts its
effects on the saliva glands, when applied to the mouth,
or even taken into the stomach ; a tincture of the bark
is good in cases of rheumatism; the substance of the
bark should be extracted by Holland gin, a table spoonful should be taken once a day ; a tincture of the berries is excellent in cases of cramp colic. The fresh
juice expressed from the roots, affords great relief in
that painful disease termed the dry belly ache. The
bark of the root dried and pulverized, is a great snuff,
to be used in cases of pain in the head, it is also good
for that painful disease called the tooth ache; it
should be put in the hollow of the tooth two or three
times a day.

WILD INDIGO, THE WEED, ROOT.

This vegetable is indigenous, and is exclusively an
American plant. It grows in great abundance in almost every barren pasture, and in woods ; the stalk
rises to two feet high, or more, sending off numerous
branches ; the leaves are small and heart shaped; it
has golden colored blossoms, which renders the plant
very conspicuous; the seed vessels are inflated, containing numerous seeds; the root is irregular in shape,
of a dark brown color externally, and sending off ma-

ny long slender branches; its taste is unpleasant — somewhat acrid, similar to that of ipecacuanha; the root, by distillation, will yield a dark blueish oil, which is very heavy and thick, and which is easily obtained by distilling. This oil is a sure remedy in cases of gravel; it acts very powerfully on the uterine vessels; it has carried off the gravel in pieces by the urine in quantities. It should be taken from three to five drops a day, in a little spicewood tea. While using of this medicine, the patient should take great care so as not to take cold; the diet should be sweetened water and bread; this course should be pursued until the patient is entirely relieved. I have never failed, with this medicine, in performing a cure. I have sent quantities of phials of this medicine, to patients who were afflicted with this complaint, in various parts of the United States, and I never have heard of its failing of performing a cure. The leaves dried, pulverized, and made into pills, is a quick and active purgative, leaving the bowels in good order.

COLTS FOOT, THE HERB AND FLOWERS.

This grows in moist situations producing yellow flowers in February and March, it is some times the case they do not flower till the last of April or the first of May, these soon fall off and are succeeded by large roundish leaves, hairy underneath, their taste is somewhat acrid, this herb is great in cases of Phthisic, and other disorders of the breast, this root boiled in new sweet milk will give immediate relief in cases of phthisic. The leaves pulverized into a powder are good in cases of Hysteric affections, particularly where it arises from a disorder of the bowels. It is also good for burning in the stomach.

The root by distillation yields an oil which is good in cases of of consumption and should be used freely in

such cases, it should be taken from twenty-five to fifty
drops two or three times a day, where the cough is bad.
When the oil is made into a tincture it is good in cases
of the mumps, half a tea sopoonful should be taken two
or three times a day in case it should fall in the testicles. The oil should be used only externally, it will
suage the inflammation in the course of a few hours
when the parts are kept warm by the fire and the application of flannel &c., this course of treatment should be
continued until a cure is obtained.

WATER PARSNIP THE HERB AND ROOT.

This is a perennial plant and grows wild by the side
of rivers and near ditches in the edge of swamps and
in dry creeks, and is found frequently in low grounds
particularly in marshy places, it resembles the tame parsnip and grows from one to two feet high the leaves are
rather more yellow than the tame parsnip. The roots
are of a whitish color, rembling calamus having joints
and being about the size of the finger, or somewhat larger, the tops of this herb boiled in new sweet milk, is
a sure remedy in cases of poison proceeding from rats-
bane, laudanum, corrosive sublimate, red precipitate or
Jamestown weed. Half a pint of this liquid should be
drank every twenty minutes until relief is obtained.—
I never have known it to fail in any of those cases.
The root pulverized, and taken in wine, is good in cases
of cutaneous affections and ulcers of all kinds; from a
table spoonful to a wine glass full, should be taken twice
or three times a day, at the same time living on light
diet.

THE COMMON BIRCH TREE.

This is a native of our country and grows in abundance on the top of cliff's, near creeks, mountains and

rivers, it is a tree very well known among the citizens in general, so that a further description is unnecessary. The inside bark of the tree pulverised and taken in French brandy is a great medicine in cases of epilepsy, it strengthens the system, purges the blood, acts on the liver and strengthens the stomach, a table spoonful may be taken two or three times a day in cases of epilepsy. The bark of the root and the body of the tree yield an essential oil, of the most stimulating nature, and is good in cases of fits, consumption and scrofula. It is also good in cases of the flour albus or diseases of the womb, particularly where there is a bearing down and burning and difficulty of making water, from twenty to thirty drops of the oil should be taken in those cases two or three times a day on a little sugar. The oil should also be rubbed on externally on the abdomen in all of those cases of female complaints of this kind.

PENNEROYAL, THE TOP.

Pennyroyal needs but little description, being so universally known, the root is annual, small, branched fibrous, and of a yellow color, the stem is from nine to fifteen inches high, the leaves are small, the flowers appear in July, and the plant continues to bloom till the last of autumn, it is distributed extensively over every part of the United States, growing always in hard dry land, it is very abundant by road sides, and the side of fences. Pennyroyal is a very powerful stimulous, the leaves boiled in strong vinegar in the form of tea, is good in cases of herpes, scald head, and any inflammation of the skin whatever. This herb by distillation yields a quantity of essential oil, which is good in cases of debility of the stomach, such as cramp colic, bilious colic and intermittent fevers, it should be used from ten to thirty drops in any of those cases, two or three times a day, it is also an excellent ointment in cases of rheumatism and callous diseases of the joints, this should be used every night and morning to the af. fected parts.

SPICE WOOD OR FEVER WOOD

This is a perennial plant of our country, and grows in swamps and near branches, it is a shrub that is universally known through the U. States. The bark of the root is excellent in cases of diarrhœa, it should be taken from ten to thirty grains in a little syrup as often as the case may require. The berries yield an essential oil by distillation, which is good in cases of dropsy of the hydro-thorax, it should be used from ten to thirty drops two or three times a day, in a little strong horsemint tea. It is also good in cases of abortion, and should be freely used in such cases, from ten to one hundred drops in a little alum water. The oil applied externally is good to heal ulcers, and is good to mix in any kind of diuretic pills,

---

GOLDEN-ROD.

This herb may be found common on pine plains, on the side of cliff's, and in hedges ; it grows about two or three feet high, has a long narrow leaf, very smooth and glossy, and a large cluster of yellow blossoms, it has a sweet spicy taste and smell resembling fennel or annis, there is also an essential oil in this herb, the blossom, leaves and root. may be distilled. This oil is good in cases of sickness at the stomach, pain in the breast, or in the side, and difficulty of breathing, colics, pains in the bowels, or pleurisy ; it should be taken in any of those cases, from ten to forty drops, three times a day in a little wine, the flowers pulverized and taken from ten to thirty grains in a little honey two or three times a day, is excellent in any kind of acute inflammation,

14

the root prepared in the same way, and taken from twenty to fifty grains two or three times a day, is good to counteract any kind of poison whatever, the leaves boiled in new sweet milk, is good for children who are subject to worms, and should be used every third or fourth night freely, the next morning after taking this tea, the child should take castor-oil sufficient to operate on the bowels, this course should be pursued with all children who are afflicted in that way.

TINCTURES.

The Tincture of Spignard, take of the oil of Spignard one ounce, the flour of benizon half an ounce, three quarts of alcohol, let it stand for three days, it is then fit for use, and should be taken from ten to thirty drops three times a day, in a little syrup or on loaf sugar, this should be taken in cases of consumption, or any debility of the lungs whatever.

The compound tincture of Horsemint — Take one ounce of the oil of horsemint, half an ounce of Balsamcopevia, half a gallon of alcohol, shake it well together, once a day for three or four days, it is then fit for use, and is good in cases of debility of the womb, particularly where there is burning and bearing down and difficulty of making water. It should be taken from a half to a tea spoonful, three times a day in a little tea of any kind, it may also be used in the same way in cases of venerial diseases.

The tincture of Dogwood berries — Take one ounce of the oil of dogwood berries, (which may be obtained by distillation,) one quart of alcohol, add them together, let it stand for two days it is then fit for use and is a great tonic in cases of debility of the stomach, particularly in dyspeptic cases, it should be taken from twelve to twenty-five drops, two or three times a day in a little water, it is also good in cases of colic taken in the same way.

The tincture of sweet fennel— Take one ounce of the oil of sweet fennel, one quart of rectified spirits, shake this well together, this is a great tincture in cases of cold or pleurisy, particularly where it is attended with a great deal of pain, hoarseness, or difficulty of breathing; a tea spoonful should be taken every half hour in a little warm coffee, until it produces a complete perspiration all over the system, the patient should avoid getting cold, the diet should also be limited.

The tincture of Calamus or sweet flag — Take of the oil of calamus one ounce, spirits of wine two quarts, let this digest for four days, this is good in cases of cramp cholic, diarrhœa and indigestion of the stomach, it may be taken from a half to a tea spoonful three times a day, according as the nature of the case may require.

The compound tincture of Musk Rat stones — Take of pulverized Musk Rat stone's, three ounces, one quart of the spirits of wine, let it digest together for ten days, this is an excellent tincture in cases of fits, and in all hysterical disorders. It should be taken from ten to thirty drops three or four times a day in a little water, in severe cases of fits it may be taken from a half to a tea spoonful three times a day.

The Compound tincture of Cinnamon.—Take of Cinnamon bark, two ounces, powdered, the same of gum-kino, one quart of rectified spirits: let it digest for five days; this is good in cases of hermorrhage, or flooding, (either from the uterus or lungs,) it should be taken from a half to a tea spoonful every two hours, until the complaint subsides; it may be taken in a little syrup.

The tincture of Spear Mint.—Take of the oil of spear mint, half an ounce, one pint of rectified spirits;

let this digest together three hours, it is good in cases of water brash, sickness at the stomach, pains in the bowels, or in pit of the stomach ; it should be taken from ten to fifty drops, three or four times a day, in a little water.

The tincture of Pennyroyal.—Take of the oil of pennyroyal one ounce, one quart of alcohol, let it digest two days, this is good in cases of chills, intermittents, cramps or coldness of any kind in the extremities. It should be taken from a half to a tea spoonful two or three times a day, or as the nature of the case may require, it may be taken in a little wine or toddy.

The tincture of Black Walnut nuts—Take four ounces of the kernels of black walnut nuts, one quart of French brandy, (the kernels should be beat fine,) let them digest together for ten days, then filter. This is good in a debilitated or deranged state of the kidneys, where it proceeds from colds, hard lifts, strains, hurts, &c. It should be taken from a half to a tea spoonful, three times a day in a little tea or wine, if it should produce an itching humor externally on the skin, a less portion may be taken.

The tincture of Paupaw seeds—Take two ounces of the seeds finely pulverized, one pint of alcohol, let them digest together for three days. This is the quickest vomit that I have ever tried. ten drops will produce vomiting in three minutes after taking it into the stomach. It is good in cases of poisons, or where anything is taken in the stomach, where it is necessary for it to be discharged from the stomach immediately, from three to four drops is a plenty for children from three to five years of age—It is a very safe emetic, though quick and powerful.

The tincture of Beech Tree nuts—Take of the oil of beech tree nuts (the oil is obtained by distillation when the nuts are ripe) half an ounce, one quart of rectified spirits, alcohol, or Holland gin, let it digest together for three days, this is a great medicine in cases of inflammation of the womb, or flour albus, or where there is an itching humor proceeding from either; from a half to a tea spoonful may be taken three times a day in a little water.

The tincture of Parsley—Take of the oil of parsley one ounce, and alcohol one quart, let it digest four days, this is good in cases of gravel, and where there is difficulty in making water. It should be taken from ten to thirty drops, three or four times a day in a little tea.

Tincture of Sassafras—Take of the oil of sassafras one ounce, of alcohol one quart, let it digest two hours, this is good in weak debilitated cases of the stomach, it is also an excellent tonic where the fevers are broken and the stomach is weak, it should be taken from ten to thirty drops three or four times a day in a little water.

The tincture of Spice wood—Take of the oil of spice wood one ounce, of French brandy half a gallon, let them digest together ten days, it is fit for use, and good to stop vomiting, purging and is a good tonic to strengthen the stomach; it should be taken from half to a tea spoonful three or four times a day, or as often as the case may require, the diet in those cases should be of a limited kind.

The tincture of Cayenne Pepper—Take cayenne one ounce, gum-myrrh four ounces, and alcohol one gallon, let them digest together five days, shaking it once or twice a day in the mean time, this may be taken in cases of pain in the stomach or bowels, and is good to relieve indigestion, looseness of the bowels—head ache, when rubbed on the face and temples and snuffed up the nose—and it is excellent to rub on externally in cases of rheumatism, incisions, or cuts, &c. The com-

mon form of taking this medicine, is in water or tea,
and may be taken in doses of from one to two tea
spoonfuls twice a day—and to use it externally, the patient must rub it on the parts affected, and repeat it as
long as it may be deemed necessary, or till relief is obtained; to take a gill of this medicince. and add one
table spoonful of the spirits of turpentine and thirty
grains of gum-camphor, this preparation well digested,
and used externally, will prove more efficacious in
rheumatisms than the above, though while applying
this last externally, the above named preparation may
be taken internally, be careful while using this medicine that you do not get wet.

The tincture of Cubebs—Take half a pound of pulverized cubebs, the same of alum, the same of refined
nitre, half a gallon of rectified spirits, let them be added together, and shook two or three times a day for ten
pays, this is a medicine in case of abortion where it
has taken place, from a half a tea spoonful may be taken
every two or three hours, as long as necessity requires
it.

The tincture of Angelica seed — Take one pound of
Angelica seed well pulverised, one pound of refined
sugar, three quarts of old rye whiskey, this should be
well shook together for five or six days, it is then fit
for use after being strained, and is good in all weak debilitated states of the system, and is a mild and pleasant
tonic, it strengthens the nerves and promotes digestion,
it may be taken from a half to a table spoonful m a little water two or three times a day.

The tincture of Beef's gall — Take of beef's gall three
ounces, the oil of angelica half an ounce, refined sugar
four ounces, the oil of tansy the fourth of an ounce,
alcohol two quarts, let it digest together five days, this
is a great preparation in cases of diseases of the gall,
where the gall ducts are stoped, it will produce that

regularity that nature requires, it will also strengthen the digestive powers of the stomach and restore the functions of the same. It should be taken from ten to forty drops two or three times a day in a little water, and repeated until the necessary relief is obtained.

The tincture of Coriander seed — Take of Coriander seed finely pulverised four ounces, one ounce of garden roses, one ounce of rhubarb, four ounces of sarsaparilla root, finely pulverized, half a gallon of rectified spirits let them digest well together ten days, it is then fit for use, and a sure remedy in cases of gonorrhœa, or clap, if taken in a short time after the infection takes place, the patient should be bled once or twice every two or three days. at the same time the bowels should be kept freely open with mild purgatives, the diet should also be very limited indeed, half a table spoonful of the tincture should be taken three times a day in a little spice tea, it is truly regretful that such a disorder should be carried too and fro through the country, yet we now and then find that such cases do occur, therefore we lay these causes down, knowing that those who have taken the contagion would be glad of relief as soon as possible — and as some of the human family are more subject to indulge themselves in the Goddess of love than some others, we deem it highly necessary to pre- scribe a remedy for those who through weakness and want of forethought and fortitude indulge therein.

The tincture of Annis — Take of the oil of annis one ounce, the fourth of an ounce of camphor, ten grains of opium, two quarts of alcohol, let them digest together for three days, this preparation is good in cases of the consumption, scrofula, or kings evil. It should be taken from ten to thirty drops three or four times a day in a little sugar, it may also be used in all weak and feeble situations of the system, &c.

The compound tincture of Mulberry—Take of the oil

of mulberry one ounce, (the oil may be obtained from the bark of the root by distillation,) one quart of recti-fied spirit, let this be well dissolved together for two days, it is then fit for use, and is a great preparation in cases of inflammatory or nervous fever, particularly where the fever appears to be confined to any one par-ticular part of the system. It acts very powerfully upon the liver and produces that regular flow of blood that is necessary, it also strengthens and acts on the nerves very powerfully, and should be freely used in such cases, it should be taken from a half to a tea spoon-ful, three or four times a day in a little tar water or tea.

The tincture of Garlic — Take of bruised garlic roots and tops one pound, French brandy two quarts, the tincture of sassafras half an ounce, half an ounce of the tincture of horse-raddish, let them digest for four days to be shook well two or three times a day, this is good in cases of cramp, bold hives, measles, &c. It should be taken two or three times a day in doses from a half to a tea spoonful, for an adult — for a child from five to ten drops, and may be taken in a little syrup or weak toddy.

The tincture of Tansy — Take of tansy one ounce, of alcohol two quarts, let them be well shook together this is good in all spasmodic affections, such as hyster-ics, cramps, colics, pleurisies from cold, it should be ta-ken from ten to fifty drops, two or three times a day in a little water and oftener if the case is urgent, it may be used with entire safety in all of those cases.

The tincture of Cloves — Take of the oil of cloves half an ounce, alcohol one quart, let it be dissolved well together, this is good in cases of bowel complaints, also flooding, it may be taken from a half to a tea spoon-ful two or three times a day, or as the case may be. In the preceeding pages I have laid down a number of tinctures which I have used advantageously in my mode of practice, though they are simple, yet they are powerful in removing disorders. Tho' they are selected out of nature's garden, they are efficacious, being planted by the wise creator for our benefit and use.— I have given each herb their common english name which is mostly used by the citizens of the country. Those preparations are mostly used among the Indians, and that with great success. When they are afflicted, they apply to the field of nature for medicine, which generally proves efficacious to them, and were we all to pursue the same course when afflicted, instead of using mineral medicines, which not only destroys the constitution, but brings on frequently a miserable life, and lastly a painful death. I am not to be understood here as speaking entirely against the proper use of mineral medicines, though I am much opposed to the quantities made use of in general, they being too much depended upon alone—when there is much better and safer remedies to be resorted to for the relief of all diseases—yet, what few I have named may be used with tolerable safety, if the directions given are strictly adhered to.

Emetics—Are medicines which excite vominting, and are usually employed in fevers of almost every species, especially when accompanied in the commencement with nausea, vomiting, and other symptoms indicating a disordered state of the stomach. They cleanse the stomach of its noxious contents, and prepare the way for the reception of the remedies.

As a general rule, emetics should always be given on an empty stomach, and in the morning. They act with greater certainty, and with less distress to the patient. They will, however, answer very well in the evening. In ordinary cases, administer the medicine in divided quantities, so as to guard against too violent an effect, and promote its operation by drinking freely of warm water. To check inordinary vomiting from too large a dose of emetic medicine, give laudanum, combined with some cordial, apply fermentations to the pit of the stomach, and sinapisms to the extremeties.

Chicken water, copiously drank, is sometimes useful, by turning the action downwards. When these fail, anodyne injections may be resorted to, and a large blister should be put on over the region of the stomach. Of the emetics, the mildest are ipecacuanha, the antimonial solution, and antimonial wine, in broken doses. The most active and expeditious, are the white and blue vitriol. Where poisons have been swallowed, one or the other of these should be given in very large doses, and repeated every fifteen minutes until the desired effect be obtained.

Antimonial solution—Take of tartar emetic six grains, water half a pint ; spirits of lavender thirty drops ; sugar, a small lump—Mix, dose for adults, a wine glassful every fifteen minutes, which should be encouraged by drinking warm water, and afterwards turned downwards by drinking gruel well salted.

Cathartics—Are medicines which by quickening the peristaltic motion, increase the evacuation of the intestines, or as may happen induce purging. Cathartics differ very materially in their degree of activity; some operating mildly, while others are more violent in their effects. The former are usually distinguished by the title of laxatives, and the latter by that of purgatives, the harshest of which, are called drastic purgatives. The primary and most obvious effect of cathartics, is the evacuation of the bowels. These are liable to various accumulations of a morbid nature, which, remaining, disturb health, and frequently excites or confirms disease. Cathartics in relieving the bowels, under such circumstances, also extend their operation upwards, and bring down in many instances, the contents of the stomach. To this may be added, that the strong impres-

sion which they impart to the liver and pancreas, ex_
cites these glands to invigorated efforts, and the result
is a vast increase of their respective secretions. It is
in this way, that congestions are removed, biliary cal_
culi dislodged, and jaundice and other affections, from
organic obstruction, cured. They also subdue the pulse,
equalize excitement, and render important service in
the management of febrile and inflammatory cases.

Exhibited in the commencement of almost any febrile
affection, they will often arrest its progress, and during
the subsequent or more advanced periods, they are
sometimes daily repeated, and so far from weakening
add to the strength of the patient.

As in the case of emetics, give the medicine on an
empty stomach, and either in the morning or at bed
time. By doing this, we prevent its being rejected,
and secure a much more easy and effectual operation.
And it should be recollected, as cathartics are of very
different properties and modes of operation, they should
be carefully selected, according to the circumstances
of the case.

Laxatives — Of this description are castor oil, sweet
oil, magesia, calomel, neutral salts, sulphur, cream of
tartar; as also the cathartic mixture, and the aperient
and diaphoretic pills, in broken doses.

Cathartic Mixture — Take of glauber salts one ounce
and a half; Lemon juice or sharp vinegar, one ounce:
water half a pint; sugar, a sufficiency to sweeten it.
Mix or take of cream of tartar finely powdered, and
manna, each one ounce: water half a pint; sugar a
sufficient quantity to sweeten it. Mix, dose for adults,
a wine glassful every hour till it operates.

Anti-bilious, or aperient and Diaphoretic pills — Take
of calomel, Jalap, each twenty grains; tartar emetic
two grains, syrup or mucilage of gum arabic sufficient
to form a mass, make eight pills. Dose for adults, two

at bed time, and the dose repeatod every hour in the morning until it operates sufficiently. Or take four in the morning, and one every hour until the desired effect be obtained.

Purgatives—The drastics are the croton-oil, gamboge, aloes, calomel, jalap, rhubarb and senna, the purgative infusion, purgative powder, stimulent purgative pills, and purgative electuary. The distinction, however, between laxatives and purgatives, is by no means easy, since by diminishing, or increasing the dose of the former they may with some propriety, be considered as belonging to the first or second class.

Purgative infusion—Take of senna and manna, each half an ounce; salts an ounce, ginger one drachm, boiling water, one pint. Dose for adults, one gill every hour or until it operates.

Purgative powder — Take of calomel and jalap, each twenty grains, to be taken in the morning in syrup or molasses by adults. Or take of rhubarb and vitriolated tartar in fine powder, each one drachm; mix well together, and divide into four powders. One taken on going to bed, and another in the morning, will be found an efficacious remedy, whenever it is required to cleanse the stomach and bowels of bilious and other offensive matter.

Stimulent purgative pills — Take of calomel, gamboge, each one drachm; syrup sufficient to form a mass. Beat them together, and then make twenty four pills. Dose for adults, from three to six. Or take of rhubarb one ounce, aloes half an ounce, calomel two drachms, syrup sufficient to form a mass, beat them well together and form pills of common size. Dose for adults from three to six. These are a most excellent pill to evacuate the superfluous matter of the stomach and bowels.

Aloetic pills — Take of aloes, in the first powder, one

drachm and a half, castile soap one drachm, ginger half a drachm — beat them well together, and then add syrup sufficient to form a mass — which is to be form. ed into forty-eight pills. Dose for adults, two at bed time, or sufficient number to keep the bowels in a reg. ular state.

Diaphoretics.—In the common langauge of schools, the term diaphoretic, is restricted to those articles on. ly, which promote the insensible perspiration; and such as occasion sweating, are distinguished by the appellation of sudorifics. But as in the medicines ar. ranged under these titles, we can discern no difference — except in the degree of force, or what arises from the manner of administration — we shall comprehend the whole under the head of diaphoretics.

To promote perspiration, it is essentially necessary that the patient should be confined to his bed. Let his pulse and the temperature of the body be carefully watched. It is a principle settled and fully recognized, never to resort to diaphoretics in fevers of an inflam. matory species, till arterial action and general excite. ment are considerably reduced by previous bleeding and evacuations, by puking or purging. After this di. rect depletion, diaphoretics then comes in with great advantage, and will commonly either mitigate or com. pletely arrest the progress of the disease.

In the exhibition of diaphoretics, give diluent drinks, unless the stomach be irritable.

This remark particularly applies to the antimonial preparations, and some of the combinations of Ipeca. cuanha. The temperature of the drinks must be regu. lated by that of the skin. The latter not being high, they should be warm, or even hot; but if the contrary prevail, they must be given cold. In the low stage of disease, while pursuing the diaphoretic plan, studi. ously avoid purging, unless circumstances imperiously require this remedy. It is very apt, in this state of the

system, to check sweating and to bring on an aggrava-
tion of the complaint.   It does this by divesting action
from the surface of the intestines, and by exposing the
patient to cold.

Diaphoretic Drops.—Take of sweet spirits of nitre
and antimonial wine, each one ounce.   Mix.   Dose for
adults, a tea spoonful every two hours.   If the stomach is in an irritable stage, add only half the quantity
of antimonial wine.

Antimonial Wine.—Dose for adults, twenty drops
every hour or two, till the proper effects be produced.

Febrifuge Powders.—Take of Ipecacuanha, two
scruples, nitre two drams; mix, and divide into twelve
doses.   One dose to be taken every two or three
hours, by adults.

Febrifuge Mixture.—Take of nitre two drachms,
lemon juice or vinegar, one ounce; water, half a pint;
sugar, a sufficient quantity to sweeten it; mix.   A
wine glass-ful to be taken by adults every two hours.
It will be rendered more active by the addition of two
drachms of antimonial wine.

Dover's Powders—Ipecacuanha, powderd, and opium, each one drachm; vitriolated tartar, in powder
one ounce.   The greatest possible pains should be taken to grind the mass to a completely fine powder.—
Nitre may be substituted for the vitriolated tartar.
when that is not at hand.   This powder is the most
efficacious sudorific we possess.
    It is an admirable remedy for quieting the bowels.
when affected by the exhibition of mercury, or any
other causes.   Doses for adults, from ten to twenty
grains every three or four hours.

Camphorated Powders—Take of camphor, two scruples; nitre, powdered, two drachms.   Moisten the

camphor with spirits, and after reducing it to a fine powder, add the nitre. Divide it into twelve doses.—One to be taken every three or four hours by adults.

Demulcent Drinks—Are those which sheath the acrimony of the humors, and render them mild, such as Flax-seed tea, marsh-mallow tea : mucilage of quince seeds. pith of sassafras, slipperyelm, and gum arabic. A solution of gum arabic is made by boiling an ounce of picked gum arabic, in a quart of water, until it be dissolved. All these are useful to sheath and defend very sensible parts from the irritation of acrid humors, as is the case in tickling-cough, and common lax, or bloody flux, heat of urine, &c., in all which, the natural mucus of the parts are defctive.

Absorbent Medicines—Are such as correct acidity in the stomach.

Calcined Magnesia—One or two tea spoonsful to be taken occasionally mixed in milk or mucilage of gum arabic, by ad.lts.

Prepared Chalk—A tea spoonful to be given in the same manner as Magnesia.

Absorbent Mixture—Take of chalk prepared, half an ounce ; gumarabic, powdered, and white sugar, each, two drachms ; water, four ounces. Dose for adults, a table spoonful every two or three hours.

Diuretics—Are remedies to promote the urinary discharges, which may take place, either by stimulating the kidneys, or by an invigoration of the powers of absorption, and especially in cases of dropsical effusions. It hence appears, that diuretics are of two species, though in which ever mode they operate, it is by an action primarily on the stomach. Extending to the absorbents or kidneys, according to the affinity of the article to the one or the other of these parts.

Mild Diuretics —Of this class of medicines, nitre, by reducing the force of circulation, will be found eminently useful in febrile cases. Dose, ten to fifteen grains, for adults, every two or three hours.

Diuretic Infusion —Pound a handful of the kernels of pumpkin seeds or melon seeds, with a small quantity of white hard sugar, to a smooth paste, then add a quart of boiling water, and a quarter of an ounce of salt petre or half an ounce of sweet spirits of nitre, and rub them well together. This is a pleasant and mild diuretic, particularly useful where the discharge of urine is attended with heat and pain. A tea cup full may be taken every hour or two by adults.

Diuretic pills — Take of dried squills in fine powder, and calomel, of each a drachm, mucilage of gum arabic sufficient to form a mass, and then make twenty pills, two of which are to be taken at bed time by adults.

These pills powerfully promotes urine, and are very efficacious in carrying off colds, &c. in dropsical swellings.

Alum — Is used in floodings, and in long continued fluxes. It is given to grown persons in doses from five to twenty grains every four, eight, or twelve hours, according to the emergency of the case. In female cases, it may commonly be used with gum-kino.

Aloes, Socotrine — Is a purgative medicine, very stimulating to the rectum or lower intestines, and if too frequently used, induces piles; it is, however, a very good article in cases of suppressed menses, worms, &c. The dose for a grown person may be from six to sixty grains; for a child two years old, the dose may be from two to six grains.

Asafœdita —Is used in hysteric cases. In hysteric suffocatlon, a plaster made of asacœdita, one quarter of an ounce, and camphor, ten to fifteen grains, may be applied to the stomach, and prove a useful remedy.

Bark—Of this article there are two kinds: that is, the red and the pale. It is a useful remedy in feeble habits, and strengthens the stomach and bowels. It is employed in the cure of the fever and ague ; but it is sometimes unsuccessful unless the patient be first bled once or twice. The dose for an adult may be from thirty to sixty grains, to be repeated every one, two, or three hours. A dose for a child of two years old, may be from five to ten grains.

Borax—Is used to relieve children of the thrush. It is also proper for making gargarisms in cases of sore throats. In cases of thrush, it may be prepared as follows: Take borax sixty grains, honey one ounce, add as much water as serves to dilute it sufficiently

It is said to be useful as a medicine to be taken inwardly in cases of flour albus. The dose from five grains to sixty ; if taken in this disease a few grains of , nutmeg or cinnamon should be added to each dose ; otherwise it may produce vomiting.

Camphor—Is a very powerful stimulent, and is sometimes useful in fevers ; after sufficient depletion it produces sweating, and may be given in doses from two to twenty grains ; it is sometimes useful combined with salt petre, when dissolved in spirits ; it is sometimes used as an external application for the relief of pain, inflammation, numbness, palsy, &c.

Carolina pink root—Perhaps the usual doses given of this medicine may be too strong ; as advised for worms ; it will be safest to make a trial as follows; take one quarter of an ounce of the pink root, stew it gently in one pint of water, down to three gills ; give half a gill of the decoction to a child of six years old, morning and evening, and observe its effects ; if it produces unusual drowsiness, the dose may be considered too

15

strong, and ought therefore, to be lessened or entirely discontinued.

Castor Oil—Is a mild and pleasant purge, a dose for an adult, is from one to two table spoonfuls; for a child of two years old and upwards, from one to two tea spoonfuls may be given.

Columbo—Is said to be almost a specific in cholera-morbus, nausea, vomiting, purging, diarrhœa. Dysentery, bilious fevers, indigestion and spasmodic stricture existing in the system, it is highly pernicious. Let it therefore be observed, that if the use of this article excites pain in the head, with other feverish symptoms, it should not be continued. It may be given in the form of simple filings, rust of iron, or the salt of steel; if the rust or filing be used, the dose may be from five to ten grains; if salt of steel be chosen, from one to three grains may be the dose; it is generally the best to administer it in small doses, frequently repeated.— Cases may occur in which this article is really necessary, and in which, notwithstanding its propriety, it may cause considerable sickness and perturbations. In such instances a moderate dose of opium may be given after each dose, or the patient may be directed to take it on going to bed at night, and again half an hour before rising up in the morning, and at other times of the day; let him or her walk moderately immediately after taking the dose, &c

Kino—Is an astringent opium, and is useful in diseases of laxity, such as diarrhœa, flux, albus, &c. It may be given in the following form: Take kino two parts, and alum three parts, grind them to powder and mix them; of this mixture, the dose may be from five to fifteen grains every three or four hours; in cases where the alum is improper or disagreeable, from five to fifteen grains of the kino alone. It may be dissolved in water, or a solution of gum arabic; to which also may be added a few drops of laudanum.

Magnesia—Is a very mild article, it corrects acidity in the stomach in its first passages; hence its effects in relieving heart burn, i. e., (burning in the stomach,) also giddiness, vomiting, and pain in the stomach, when they are the consequences of an acrid matter collected in the stomach; it also relieves gripes in children, when brought on by the same cause; a dose for an infant, may be from two to five grains, to be given in a tea of fennel seed, and repeated; the addition of a small portion of rhubarb or manna, gives it a little more activity as a purge.

Manna—Is one of the mildest purgatives, and may be given with great safety to children, and pregnant women; it is proper in pleurisy, all inflammatory fevers, and such other cases as may require mild purges. Its doses are from half an ounce to two ounces, and it is best perhaps, to dissolve it in a decoction of cassia, which is an inferior kind of cinnamon; if a litttle tartar emetic, or some other article be added, the manna will operate much more effectual—say manna half an ounce, tartar emetic half a grain, to be repeated every two or three hours. This would be an excellent preparation as a purge in child bed fever.

Gum-Myrrh—Is a stimulating medicine, and is admissable in those cases only where iron is proper, as in chlorosis: and a dose may be from five to thirty grains; a tincture may be made of this gum, as follows: Take gum-myrrh, three ounces, proof spirits, or good wine, one pint and a half, digest them ten days, with a gentle heat; the tincture so prepared is a useful addition to cleaning gargarisms, such as are proper in putrid sore throats.

Nutmeg—Warm and agreeable to the taste, is good for the stomach, corrects a laxative habit, relieves indigestion; a dose is from six to thirty grains; if roasted in substance, it is said to be more astringent, and is an excellent remedy in chronic diarrhæas and dysenteries.

Orange-peel—Is employed as a stomachic medicine, it promotes appetite, gives strength and vigor to the bowels; and is therefore, proper in cases of indigestion, flatulency, debility, &c. It is rendered more effectual by joining it with columbo: the yellow outside rhine should be preferred; infusions with water are better than any preparation with ardent spirits, in all cases where bitters are required, the use of spirits must be injurious; wine, if good, might be useful.

Olive Oil—Also called Sweet oil, is employed as an external application; it is improper, however, in cases of burns, especially if the skin peel off; but I intend, in a particular manner, to recommend a frequent use of it internally, to such women as are wont to have hard labors; they should begin its use several days before the time of delivery; one or two ounces should be beaten up with one or more yolks of an egg, till it will readily mix with water, add half a pint or a pint of water sweetened with manna, or syrup; with this she should keep her bowels constantly laxed; where there is sufficient strength, blood letting should also be employed·

Opium—Is a powerful cordial, it eases pain, but at the same time, very much increases the circulation, and is, therefore, very injurious in inflammatory fevers, especially if the brain, lungs, liver, stomach or bowels, be the seat of the disease, at least considerable evacuation should be procured, before it is ever employed; in such cases it is never proper, if there be tensity in the pulse; in cases of external tumor, and consequent pain it is frequently admissable; and when debility prevails with

a soft and languid pulse, it is an excellent remedy. Its doses when taken in substance, may be from one to three grains, in a liquid form ; as laudanum or tincture of opium, which are two different names, for the same thing; the dose may be from twenty-five to sixty drops: but it should be remembered, that this article generally produces costiveness.

Rhubarb—Is a mild purge, and may be given in do. ses of from twenty to sixty grains, but as it is considera. bly astringent, it sho'd not be employed where a costive habit is to be avoided in chronic diarrhæas, it may be giv- en in small doses of five or six srains combined with opi. um, two or three times a day ; it cannot be a proper remedy in inflammatory cases, and is therefore, forbid. den in dysentery; but in case of debility, it is frequent. ly useful ; combined with manna it will evacuate the intestines without exhausting the strength of the pa- tient in any considerable degree.

Russian Castor—Is useful in hysteric cases ; this may also be used in form of a tincture: Take castor one ounce, proof spirits one quart, digest ten days, and it is ready for use ; the dose may be from twenty to sixty drops; it is sometimes taken to advantage in conjunction with laudanum—say laudanum twenty to sixty drops, tincture of castor twenty-five drops, the whole for one dose in hysteric suffocation, as also in painful menstruation, where blood letting is not needed.

Sal-Ammoniac—Of this, one ounce may be dissolved in one quart of water, or of spirits and water combined. This solution is useful as an external application in ca- ses of inflamed breasts.

Spirits of nitre or ether—Is used in fever, and is an excellent medicine for quenching thirst, expelling flat- ulencies, preventing nausea and vomiting, and mode- rately strengthening the stomach ; it is diaphoretic and cooling. The dose may be from thirty to forty drops.

Spirits of Sal-ammoniac and spirits of harts-horn—

Are similar in their nature and effects, but the first is perhaps the best; the dose may be from fifteen to sixty drops. It is useful in fainting, and other hysteric affections; if given in wine-whey, it generally produces a very pleasant sweat.

Salt petre, also called nitre—Is a useful remedy in inflammatory fever; the dose varies from three to forty grains, every three hours; it is most effectual if given immediately after its solution. Some caution however, is necessary in using articles, as it sometimes occasions a nausea, or pain in the stomach; in such cases it requires plentiful dilution, and sometimes the addition of a little camphor. Nitre is an excellent ingredient in gargarisms, and mouth waters.

Salt of tartar, called also fixed alkali—Is used for making the saline mixture. Take salt of tartar twenty grains, lime juice or vinegar, as much as will saturate it, or till it ceases effervescence, pure water one and a half ounces, and syrup two ounces: the whole may be taken in the course of four hours, to be repeated as often as may be thought necessary, it may be given also in a simple solution with pure water, in this shape the dose may be from ten to thirty grains; but it should also be sufficiently diluted; every three or four grains requires an ounce of water. The saline mixture given in a state of effervescence will frequently correct vomiting. The simple solution of tartar relieves heart-burns, &c.

Senna—It is a purge of considerable activity; is commonly taken in form of an infusion; pour one pint of boiling water, on one quarter of an ounce of senna; let it stand severl hours in a moderate degree of heat: one gill may be taken every three hours as a dose for a grown person, and one or two spoonsful for a child two years old. It is rendered more pleasant and mild in its operation, if one ounce of manna he added: the

addition of a small portion of ginger will (help to) prevent its griping.

Flour of Sulphur—Is a gentle and pleasant purge;
it is also effectual in curing affections of the skin, as
the itch, &c. Combined with the cream of tartar, it is
useful in the piles; it is also a very good purge to be
employed on the third and fourth days of the measles.

SURGERY.

Broken bone's limbs, &c—As I do not profess surgery, I will make but a few remarks on that subject. I
have discovered a great lack in surgery, in giving directions and medicines to their patients in such cases. It
should be strictly understood, that nature is the grand
physician to cure bones as well as the flesh, that when
a bone is broken and set by any person, the diet should
be regulated and the blood calmed by proper means to
keep the wound from inflaming or getting humorish,
which will be a means of preventing mortification with
other consequences. This great lack may not be universal, but it prevails to a great extent. I would rather venture a common skillful person to set a bone by
feeling round the limb to place the bones together, and
give proper directions for medicines and diet, than to
venture a professed doctor to do it, and give no directions to regulate the blood.

Directions for broken bones, bruises, &c—Give three
doses a day of No. 1, and see that the patient is g
into a moist sweat once a day. When a bruise is first
received, bathe the part in cold vinegar and salt, or
cold water, rubbing the part severely for 30 minutes,

and if very bad, bleed the person as near the wound as convenient, and as soon as possible ; and after an hour or so, warm your vinegar and dissolve salt in it as long as it will dissolve, and bathe the part repeatedly with it as hot as they can bear it, and at intervals keep a cloth wet with it applied to the place. This should be done whenever we suppose there is bruised blood in the system, from wounds and the like, get the person into a moist sweat, and keep it up as steady as possible to keep off inflammation, and if inflammation has ensued, follow the same rule if the bone is broken. You may apply these means without rubbing that part after the bone is set.

If you undertake to set a bone or joint that has slipped, grst apply warm water round the place to loosen the cords, then place your bones by feeling around— give diet No. 2 during the whole time, till the difficulty or danger is over ; then rise to No. 3 till well. Apply medicine No. 6 to the place, or as near it as possible, during the time. A bone ought to be kept very still till it has time to knit together. If the wound should be such as to confine the patient so that they cannot exercise, they ought to have a dose or two of castor-oil to keep the bowels regular in their discharge. These directions may be applied to all the receipts for wounds that are in substance. The following are taken in part from McKenzie's Receipts.

If, in consequence of a broken bone or other injury, the patient is unable to walk, take a door from its hinges, lay him carefully on it, and have him carried by assistants to the nearest house. If no door or sofa can be procured, two boards, sufficiently long and broad, should be naild to two cross pieces, the ends of which must project about a foot, so as to form handles. If in the woods, or where no boards can be procured, a litter may be formed from the branches of trees. In this way a hand-barrow may be constructed in a few minutes, on which the sufferer may be properly carried.

If he has been wounded and bleeds, the bleeding must be stopped before he is removed.

Having reached a house, lay him on a bed, and undress him with care and gentleness. If any difficulty arises in getting off his coat or pantaloons, rip up the seams, rather than use force. This being done, proceed to ascertain the nature of the injury.

This may be either simple or compound ; that is, it may be a contusion or bruise, a wound, fracture, or dislocation, or it may be two or all of them united in one or several parts.

A contusion is the necessary consequence of every blow, and is known by the swelling and discoloration of the skin.

Wounds are self-evident.

Fractures are known by the sudden and severe pain, by the misshapen appearance of the limb, sometimes by its being shortened, by the patient being unable to move it without excruciating pain, but most certainly, by grasping the limb above and below the spot where the fracture is supposed to exist, and twisting it different ways, when a grating will be felt, occasioned by the broken ends of the bone rubbing against each other. If the swelling, however, is very great, the experiment should not be made until it it reduced.

Dislocations, or bones being out of joint, are known by the deformity of the joint when compared with its fellow, by the pain and inability to move the limb, by its being longer or shorter than usual, and by the impossibility of moving it in praticular directions.

The most serious effects, however, resulting from contusions, are when the blow is applied to the head, producing either concussion or compression of the brain.

Concussion of the brain. Symptoms—The patient is stunned, his breathing low, drowsiness, stupidity, the the pupil of the eye rather contracted, vomiting. After a time he recovers.

Treatment—Apply cloths dipped in cold vinegar and salt to his head, and when the stupor is gone, bleed him and open his bowels with epsom salts. He should be confined to bed, in a quiet situation, and every measure taken to prevent an inflammation of the brain, which, if it comes on, must be treated by copious bleeding, and bathe with vinegar and salt.

Compression of the brain. Symptoms—Loss of sense and motion, slow, noisy and laborious breathing, pulse slow and irregular, the muscles relaxed, as in a person just dead, the pupil of the eye enlarged, and will not contract even by a strong light, the patient lies like one in an apoplectic fit, and cannot be roused.

Treatment—Shave the head, and if possible, procure surgical assistance without delay, as there is nothing but an operation can be of any avail.

For management, see 207th page.

Of Wounds--Wounds are of three kinds, viz: incised, punctured and contused ; among the latter are included gun-shot wounds. The first step in all wounds is

To stop the bleeding—If the flow of blood is but trifling, draw the edges of the wound together with your hand, and hold them in that position some time, when it will frequently stop. If, on the contrary, it is large, of a bright red color, flowing in spirts or with a jerk, clap your finger on the spot it springs from, and hold it there with a firm pressure, while you direct some one to pass a handkerchief round the limb (supposing the wound to be in one) above the cut, and to tie its two ends together in a hard knot. A cane, whip-handle, or stick of any kind, must now be passed under the knot, (between the upper surface of the limb and the handkerchief,) and turned round and round until the the stick is brought down to the thigh, so as to make the handkerchief encircle it with considerable tightness.

You may then take off your finger, if the blood still flows, tighten the handkerchief by a turn or two of the stick, until it ceases. The patient may now be removed (taking care to secure the stick in its position) without running any risk of bleeding to death by the way.

Eor management, refer to page 207·

As this apparatus cannot be left on for any length of time, without destroying the life of the part, endeavor as soon as possible to secure the bleeding vessels, and take it off. Having waxed together three or four threads of sufficient length, cut the ligature they form, into as many pieces as you think there are vessels to be taken up, each piece being about a foot long. Wash the parts with warm water, and then with a sharp hook, or a slender pair of pincers in your hand, fix your eye steadfastly upon the wound, and direct the handkerchief to be relaxed by a turn or two of the stick: you will now see the mouth of the artery from which the blood springs; seize it with your hook or pincers, draw it a little out, while some one passes a ligature round it, and ties it up tight with a double knot. In this way take up in succession every bleeding vessel you can see or get hold of.

If the wound is too high up in a limb to apply the handkerchief, don't lose your presence of mind, the bleeding can still be commanded. If it is the thigh, press firmly in the groin; if in the arm, with the hand or ring of a common door key, make pressure above the collar bone, and about the middle against the first rib which lies under it. The pressure is to be continued until assistance is procured, and the vessel tied up.

If the wound is on the head, press your finger firmly on it. until a compress can be brought, which must be bound firmly over the artery by a bandage.— If the wound is in the face, or so situated that pressure cannot be effectually made, or you cannot get hold of the vessel, and the blood flows fast, place a piece of ice directly over the wound, and let it remain there till

the blood coagulates, when it may be removed, and a
compress and a bandage be appplied.

For management, cite to page 207.

Incised Wounds—By an incised wound is meant a
clean cut. Having stopped the bleeding, wash away
all the dirt, &c., that may be in it with a sponge and
warm water, then draw the sides of the wound together, and keep them in that position by narrow strips of
sticking plaster, placed on at regular distances, or from
one to two inches apart. A soft compress of old linen
or lint may be laid over the whole.

Should much inflammation follow, remove the strips,
sweat and bathe the patient, (with salt and vinegar) who
should live very low, and be kept perfectly quiet according to the exigency of the case. If it is plain that
matter must form before the wound will heal, apply
No. 6, until that event takes place.

Although narrow strips of linen, spread with sticking plaster, or No. 6, form the best means of keeping
the sides of a wound together, when they can be applied, yet in the ear, nose, tongue, lips, and eye-lids, it
is necessary to use stitches, which are made in the following manner: Having armed a common needle
with a double waxed thread, pass the point of it through
the skin, at a little distance from the edge of the cut,
and bring it out of the opposite one at the same distance. If more than one stich is required, cut off the
needle, thread it again, and proceed as before, until a
sufficient number are taken, leaving the threads loose
until all the stitches are passed, when the respective
ends of each thread must be tied in a hard double knot,
drawn in such a way that it bears a little on the side
of the cut. When the edges of the wound are partly
united by inflammation, cut the knots carefully, and
withdraw the threads.

From what has been said, it must be evident that in
all wounds, after arresting the flow of blood, and

cleansing the parts, if necessary, the great indication is to bring their sides into contact throughout their whole depth, in order that they may grow together as quick. ly as possible, and without the intervention of any matter. To obtain this very desirable result, in addition to the means already mentioned, there are two things to be attended to, the position of the patient and the appli. cation of the bandage. The position of the patient should be such as will relax the skin and muscles of the part wounded, thereby diminishing ther tendency to separate.

A common bandage of a proper width, passed over the compresses moderately tight, not only serves to keep them in their place, but also tends by its pressure to forward the great object already mentioned. If, however, the wound is so extensive and painful that the limb or body of the patient cannot be raised for the purpose of applying or removing it, the best way is to spread the two ends of one or two strips of linen or leather with sticking plaster, which may be applied in place of the bandage, as follows: attach one end of a strip of the sound skin, at a short distance from the edge of the compress, over which it is to be drawn with moderate firmness and secured in a similar man- ner on its opposite side. A second or third may, if necessary, be added in the same way.

Punctured Wounds—These are caused by sharp pointed instruments, as needles, awls, nails, &c. Hav- ing stopped the bleeding, withdraw any foreign body, as part of a needle, bit of glass, &c., that may be in it, provided it can be done easily : and if enlarging the wound a little will enable you to succeed in this, do so. Though it is not always necessary to enlarge wounds of this nature, yet in hot weather it is a mark of pre- caution, which should never be omitted. As soon as this is done, pour a little turpentine into the wound or touch it with caustic, and then cover it with No. 6.

This practice may prevent the lock-jaw, which is but too frequent a consequence of wounds of this description.

Contused Wounds—Wounds of this nature are caused by round or blunt bodies, as musket balls, clubs, stones, &c. They are in general attended by but little bleeding; if, however, there should be any, it must be stopped. If it arises from a ball which can be easily found and withdrawn, it is proper to do so, as well as any piece of the clothing, &c., that may be in it; or if the ball can be distinctly felt directly under the skin, make an incision across it, and take it out, but never allow of any poking in the wound to search for such things: the best extractor of them, as well as the first and best application in contused wounds, proceed from what they may, being a soft bread and milk poultice.

If the wound is much torn, wash the parts very nicely with warm water, and then (having secured every bleeding vessel) lay them all down in as natural a position as you can, draw the edges gently together, or as much so as possible, by strips of sticking plaster, or stitches if necessary. A soft poultice is to be applied over the whole, or No. 6.

Wounds of the Ear, Nose, &c—Wash the parts clean, and draw the edges of the wound together by as many stitches as are necessary. If the part is even completely separated, and has been trodden under feet, by washing it in warm water, and placing it accurately in the proper place by the proper means, it will adhere.

Wounds of the Scalp—In all wounds of the scalp, it is necessary to shave off the hair. When this is done, wash the parts well, and draw the edges of the wound together with sticking plaster. If it has been violently torn up in several pieces, wash and lay them all down on the skull again, drawing their edges as nearly together as possible, by sticking plaster, or, if necessary, by stitches. Cover the whole with a soft compress, smeared with some simple ointment, or No. 6.

For management, refer to page 207.

Wounds of the Throat—Seize and tie up every bleeding vessel you can get hold of. If the wind-pipe is cut only partly through, secure it with sticking plaster. If it is completely divided, bring its edges together by stitches, taking care to pass the needle through the loose membrane that covers the wind-pipe itself. The head should be bent on the breast, and and secured by bolsters and bandages in that position, to favor the approximation of the edges of the wound.

Wounds of the Chest—If it is a simple incised wound, draw the edges of it together by sticking plaster, cover it over with a compress of linen, or No. 6, and pass a bandage round the chest. The patient is to be confined to his bed.

Should it be occasioned by a bullet, extract it, and any pieces of cloth, &c., that may be lodged in it, if possible, and cover the wound with a piece of linen, smeared with some simple ointment, or No. 6, taking care that it is not drawn into the chest. If a portion of the lung protrudes, return it without any delay, but as gently as possible,.

Wounds of the Belly—Close the wound by strips of sticking plaster, and stitches passed through the skin, about half an inch from its edges, and cover the whole with soft compress, secured by a bandage.

Should any part of the bowels come out at the wound, if clean and uninjured, return it as quickly as possibe: if covered with dirt, clots of blood, &c, wash it carefully in warm water, previous to so doing. If the gut

is wounded, and only cut partly through, draw the two
edges of it together by a stich. and return it; if completely divided, connect the edges by four stitches at
equal distances, and replace it in the belly, always leaving the end of the ligature projecting from the external
wound, which must be closed by sticking plaster. In
five or six days, if the threads are loose, withdraw
them gently and carefully.

For management, see page 207.

Wounds of Tendons—Tendons, or sinews, are frequently wounded, or ruptured. They are to be treated
precisely like any other wound, by keeping their divided parts together. The tendon which connecs the
great muscle forming the calf of the leg, with the heel,
called the tendon of Achilles, is frequently cut with the
adze, and ruptured in jumping from heights. This accident is to be remedied by drawing up the heel, extending the foot, and placing a splint on the fore part
of the leg, extending from the knee to beyond the
toes, which being secured in that position by a bandage, keep the foot in the position just mentioned.—
The hollows under the splint must be filled up with tow
or cotton. If the skin falls into the space between the
ends of the tendon, apply a piece of sticking plaster,
so as to draw it out of the way. It takes five or six
weeks to unite, but no weight should be laid on the
limb for several months.

Of Fractures—The signs by which fractures may
known, having been already pointed out with sufficient
minuteness, it will be unnecessary to dwell thereon; it
will be well, however, to recollect this general rule. In
cases where, from the accompanying circumstances and
symptoms, a strong suspicion exists that the bone is
fractured, it is proper to act as though it were positive-
ly ascertained to be so.

Fracture of the Bone of the Nose—The bones of the

nose, from their exposed situation, are frequently forced in. Any smooth article that will pass into the nostril, should be immediately introduced with one hand, to raise the depressed portions to the proper level, while the other is employed in moulding them into the required shape.

Fracture of the Lower Jaw.—This accident is easily discovered by looking into the mouth, and is to be remedied by keeping the lower jaw firmly pressed against the upper one, by means of a bandage passed under the chin and over the head. If it is broken near the angle, or that part nearest the ear, place a cushion or roll of linen in the hollow behind it, over which the bandage must pass, so as to make it push that part of the bone forward. The parts are to be confined this way for twenty days, during which time, all the nourishment that is taken should be sucked between the teeth. If, in consequence of the blow, a tooth is loosened, do not meddle with it, for if let alone, it will grow fast again.

Fracture of the Collar Bone—This accident is a very common occurrence, and is known at once by passing the finger along it, and by the swelling, &c. To reduce it, seat the patient in a chair without any shirt, and place a pretty stout compress of linen, made in the shape of a wedge, under his arm, the thick end of which should press against the arm-pit. His arm, bent to a right angle at the elbow, is now to be brought down to his side, and secured in that position by a long bandage, which passes over the arm of the affected side and round the body. The fore-arm is to be supported across the breast by a sling. It takes from four to five weeks to re-unite.

Fractures of the Arm. Seat the patient on a chair,

16

or the side of a bed, let one assistant hold the sound
arm, while another grasps the wrist of the broken one,
and steadily extend it in an opposite direction, bending
the fore-arm a little to serve as a lever.   You can now
place the bones in their proper situation.   Two splints
of shingle or stout paste board, long enough to reach
from below the shoulder to near the elbow, must then
be well covered with tow or cotton, and laid along
each side of the arm, and kept in that position by a bandage.   The fore-arm is to be supported in a sling.
Two smaller splints may for better security be laid between the first ones, that is one on top, and the other
underneath the arm, to be secured by the bandage in
the same way as the other.

Fractures of the Bones of the Fore-Arm.   These are
to be reduced precisely in the same way, excepting the
mode of keeping the upper portion of it steady, which
is done by grasping the arm above the elbow.   When
the splints and bandage are applied, support it in a sling.

Fractures of the Wrist.   This accident is of rare occurrence.   When it does happen the injury is generally so great as to require amputation.   If you think the
hand can be saved, lay it on a splint well covered with
tow; this extends beyond the fingers; place another
splint opposite to it, lined with the same soft material,
and secure them by a bandage.   The hand is to be carried in a sling.

The bones of the hand are sometimes broken.   When
this is the case, fill the palm with soft compresses or
tow, and then lay a splint on it, long enough to extend
from the elbow to beyond the ends of the fingers, to be
secured by a bandage, as usual.

When a finger is broken extend the end of it until it
becomes straight, place the fractured portion in its place,
and then apply two small pasteboard splints, one below
and the other above, to be secured by a narrow band-

age. The top splint should extend from the end of the finger over the back of the hand. It may sometimes be proper to have two additional splints for the sides of the finger.

Fractures of the Ribs. When, after a fall or blow, the patient complains of a pricking in his side, we may suspect a rib is broken. It is ascertained by placing the tips of two or three fingers on the spot where the pain is, and desire the patient to cough, when the grating sensation will be felt. All that is necessary, is to pass a broad bandage round the chest, so tight as to prevent the motion of the ribs in breathing; and apply No. 6 over the place.

Fractures of the Thigh. This bone is frequently broken, and hitherto has been considered the most difficult of all fractures to manage. To the ingenuity, however, of Dr. Hartshorne, the world is indebted for an apparatus which does away the greatest impediments that have been found to exist in treating it, so as to leave a straight limb without lameness or deformity; nor is it the least of its merits, that any man of common sense can apply it nearly as well as a surgeon.

It consists of two splints, made of half or three-quarter inch well seasoned stuff, from eight to ten inches wide, one of which should reach from a little above the hip, to fifteen or sixteen inches beyond the foot, while the other extends the same length from the groin. The upper end of the inner splint is hollowed out and well padded or stuffed. Their lower ends are held together by a cross piece, having two tenons, which enter two vertical mortices, one in each split, and secured there by pins. In the centre of this cross piece (which should be very solid) is a female screw. Immediately above the vertical mortices, are two horizontal ones of considerable length, in which slides the tenons of a second cross piece, to the upper side of which is fastened a foot block, shaped like the sole of a shoe, while in the other is a round hole for the reception of the head of the male screw, which passes through the female one just noticed. On the top of this cross piece — to which the foot block is attached — are two pins, which fall into grooves at the head of the screw, thereby firmly connecting them. The foot block, as before observed, is shaped like the sole of a shoe. Near the toe is a slit, through which passes a strap and buckle. Near the heel are a couple of straps, with two rings, arranged precisely like those of a skate, of which, in fact, the whole foot block is an exact resemblance. A long male screw, of wood or other material, completes the apparatus.

To apply it, put a slipper on the foot of the broken limb, and lay the apparatus over the broken leg. By turning the screw, the foot block will be forced up to the foot in the slipper, which is to be firmly strapped to it, as boys fasten their skates. By turning the screw the contrary way, the padded extremity of the inner splint presses against the groin, and the foot is gradually drawn down, until the broken limb becomes of its natural length and appearance, when any projection or inequality that may remain, can be felt and reduced by a gentle pressure of the hand.

The great advantages of this apparatus, I again repeat, are the ease with which it is applied, and the certainty with which it acts. The foot once secured to the block — in a way that every school boy understands — nothing more is required than to turn the screw until the broken limb is found to be of the same length as the sound one. It is right to observe that this should not be effected at once, it being better to turn the screw a little every day, until the limb is sufficiently extended.

As this apparatus may not always be at hand, it is proper to mention the next best plan of treating the accident. It is found in the splints of Desault, improved by Dr. Physic, consisting of four pieces. The first has a crutch head, and extends from the arm pit, to six or eight inches beyond the foot. A little below the crutch are two holes, and near the lower end, on the inside, is a block, below which there is also a hole. The second reaches from the groin, the same length with the first, being about three inches wide above, and two below. Two pieces of stout pasteboard, as many handkerchiefs or bands of muslin, with some tow and a few pieces of tape, form the catalogue of the apparatus.

It is applied as follows : Four or five pieces of tape are to be laid across the bed, at equal distances from each other. Over the upper two, is placed one of the short pasteboard splints, well covered with tow. The patient is now to be carefully and gently placed on his back, so that his thigh may rest on the splint. One of the handkerchiefs, or a strong soft band, is to be passed between the testicle and thigh of the affected side, and its ends held by an assistant, standing near the head of the bed. The second handkerchief is to be passed round the ankle, crossed on the instep and tied under the sole of the foot. By steadily pulling these two handkerchiefs, the limb is to be extended, while, with the hand, the broken bones are replaced in their natural position. The long splint is now to be placed by the side of the patient, the crutch in the arm-pit, (which is defended with tow,) while the short one is laid along the inside of the thigh and leg. The ends of the first handkerchief—being passed through the upper holes— are to be drawn tight and secured by a knot, while the ends of the second pass over the block before mentioned to be fastened in like manner at the lower one. All that remains is the short pasteboard splint, which being well covered with tow, is to be laid on the top of the thigh. The tape being tied so as to keep the four splints together, completes the operation.

Tow is to be every where interposed between the splints and the limb, and a large handful of it placed in the groin, to prevent irritation from the upper or counter extending band. It is necessary to be careful, while tying the two handkerchiefs, that they are not relaxed, so that if the operation is properly performed, the two limbs will be nearly of an equal length.

The superior advantages of Hartshorne's apparatus over this, as well as all others, must be evident to every one acquainted with the difficulty of keeping up that constant extension which is so absolutely necessary to avoid deformity and lameness, and which is so completely effected by the screw. Next to that, however, stands the one just described, which can be made by any carpenter in a few minutes, and which, if carefully applied, will be found to answer well.

Fractured thighs and legs generally re-unite in six or eight weeks ; in old men, however, they require three or four months.

In cases of fracture of the thigh or leg, the patient should always, if possible, be laid on a matrass supported by boards instead of the sacking, which, from its elasticity and the yielding of the cords, is apt to derange the position of the limb.

Fractures of the Knee Pan—This accident is easily ascertained on inspection. It may be broken in any direction, but is most generally so, across or transversely. It is reduced by bringing the fragments together, and keeping them in that position by a long bandage passed carefully round the leg, from the ankle to the knee, then pressing the upper fragment down so as to meet its fellow, (the leg being extended,) and placing a thick compress of linen above it, over which the bandage is to be continued.

The extended limb is now to be laid on a broad splint, extending from the buttock to the heel, thickly covered with tow to fill up the inequalities of the leg. For additional security, two strips of muslin may be nailed to the middle of the splint, and one on each side, and passed about the joint, one below, and the other above, so as to form a figure of eight. In twenty or thirty days the limb should be moved a little to prevent stiff. ness.

If the fracture is through its length, bring the parts together, place a compress on each side, and keep them together, with a bandage, leaving the limb extended and at rest. Any inflammation in this, or other fracture, is to be combatted by bleeding, &c.

Fracture of the Leg—From the thinness of the parts covering the principal bone of the leg, it is easy to ascertain if it is broken obliquely. If, however, the fracture be directly across, no displacement will occur, but the pain, swelling, and the grating sensation, will sufficiently decide the nature of the accident.

If the fracture is oblique, let two assistants extend the limb, while the broken parts are placed by the hand in their natural position. Two splints, that reach from a little above the knee to nine or ten inches below the foot, having near the upper end of each four holes, and a vertical mortice near the lower end, into which is fitted, a cross piece, are now to be applied as follows : Lay two pieces of tape about a foot long, on each side of the leg, just below the knee joint, and secure them there by several turns of a bandage ; pass a silk handkerchief round the ankle, cross it on the instep, and tie it under the sole of the foot. The two splints are now placed one on each side of the leg, the four ends of the pieces of tape passed through the four holes and firmly tied, and the cross piece placed in the mortice. by tying the ends of the handkerchief to the cross piece the business is finished.

If the fracture is across, and no displacement exists, apply two splints of stout pasteboard, reaching from the heel to the knee, and well covered with tow, one on each side of the leg, securing them by a bandage passing round the limb, and outside the splints.

In cases of oblique fractures of the leg close to the

knee, Hartshorne's apparatus for fractured thighs should
be applied, as already directed.

Fractures of the Bones of the Foot—The bone of the
heel is sometimes, though rarely, broken.   It is known
by a crack at the moment of the accident, a difficulty
of standing, by the swelling, and by the grating noise
on moving the heel.   To reduce it, take a long bandage, lay the end of it on the top of the foot, carry it
over the toes under the sole, and then by several turns
secure it in that position.

The foot being extended as much as possible, carry
the bandage along the back of the leg above the knee,
where it is to be secured by several turns. and then
brought down on the front of the leg, to which it is secured by circular turns.   In this way the broken pieces
will be kept in contact, and in the course of a month
or six weeks will be united.

Fractures of the foot, toes, &c., are to be treated
like those of the hand and fingers.

Of Dislocations—The signs by which a dislocation
may be known, have been already mentioned.   It is
well to recollect that the sooner the attempt is made to
reduce it, the easier it will be done.   The strength of
one man, properly applied, at the moment of the accident, will often succeed in restoring the head of a bone
to its place, which in a few days would have required
the combined efforts of men and pulleys.   If after
several trials with the best apparatus that can be mus-
tered, you find you cannot succeed, make the patient
drink strong hot tody of brandy or other spirits, until
he is very drunk.   In this way owing to the relaxed
state of the muscles, a very slight force will often be
sufficient, where a very great one has been previously
used without effect.

If any objections are made to this proceeding, or if
the patient will not consent to it, having your appara-

tus (which is presently to be mentioned) all ready, make him stand up, and bleed him in that position until he faints; the moment this happens, apply your extending and counter-extending forces. Another important rule is, to vary the direction of the extending force.— A slight pull in one way will often effect what has been in vain attemated by greater force in another.

Dislocation of the Lower Jaw. This accident, which is occasioned by blows, or yawning, is known by an inability to shut the mouth and the projection of the chin, To reduce it, seat the patient in a chair with his head supported by the breast of an assistant, who stands behind him. Your thumbs being covered with leather, are then to be pushed between the jaws, as far back as possible, while with the fingers, outside, you grasp the bone, which is to be pressed downwards, at the same time that the chin is raised. If this is properly done, the bone will be found moving when the chin is to be pushed backwards, and the thumbs slipped between the jaws and the cheeks. If this is not done, they will oe bitten by the sudden snap of the teeth as they come together, The jaws should be kept closed by a bandage for a few days.

Dislocation of the Collar Bone. This bone is rarely dislocated. Should it occur, apply the bandage, &c. directed for a fracture of the same part.

Dislocation of the Shoulder. Dislocations of the shoulder are the most common of all accidents of the kind. It is very easily known by the deformity of the joint, and the head of the bone being found in some unnatural position. To reduce it, seat the patient in a chair, place one band on the prominent part of the shoulder blade, just above the spot where the head of the bone should be, while with the other you grasp the arm above the elbow and pull it outwards.

Should this not succeed, lay the patient on the ground, place your heel in the arm-pit, and steadily and forcibly extend the arm, by grasping it at the wrist. The same thing may he tried in various positions, as placing yourself on the ground with him, laying him on a low bed while you are standing near the foot of it, &c.

If this fails, pass a strong band over the shoulder, carry it across the breast, give the ends to assistants, or fasten them to a staple in the wall; the middle of a strong band or folded towel is now to be laid on the arm above the elbow, and secured there by numerous turns of the bandage. The two ends of the towel being then given to assistants, or connected with a pulley, a steady, continued, and forcible extension is to be made, while with your hands you endeavor to push the head of the bone into its place.

Dislocation of the Elbow. If the patient has fallen on his hands, or holds his arm bent at the elbow, and every endeavor to straighten it gives him pain, it is dislocated backwards. Seat him in a chair, let one person grasp the arm near the shoulder, and another the wrist, and forcibly extend it, while you interlock the fingers of both hands just above the elbow, and pull it backwards, remembering that under those circumstances, whatever degree of force is required, should be applied in this direction. The elbow is sometimes dislocated sideways or laterally. To reduce it, make extension by pulling at the wrist, while some one secures the arm above, then push the bone into its place either inwards or outwards, as may be required. After the reduction of a dislocated elbow, keep the joint at perfect rest for five or six days, and then move it gently. If inflammation comes on, for management, see page 207.

Dislocation of the Wrist, Fingers, &c. Dislocation of the wrists, fingers, and thumb, are readily perceived on examination ; they are all to be reduced by forcibly extending the lower extremity of the part, and pushing the bones into their place. If necessary, small bands may be secured to the fingers by a narrow bandage, to facilitate the extension. These accidents should be at. tended to without delay, for if neglected for a little time, they become irremediable.

Dislocation of the Thigh. Notwithstanding the hip joint is the strongest one in the body, it is sometimes dislocated. As a careful examination of the part, com. paring the length and appearance of the limb with its fellow, &c, sufficiently mark the nature of the accident, we will proceed to state the remedy.

Place the patient on his back, upon a table covered with a blanket. Two sheets, folded like cravats, are then to be passed between the thigh and testicle of each side, and their ends (one half of each sheet pass. ing obliquely over the belly to the opposite shoulder, while the other half passes under the back in the same direction) give to several assistants. or what is much better, tied very firmly to a hook, staple, post, or some immoveable body. A large, very strong napkin, folded as before, like a cravat, is now to be laid along the top of the thigh so that its middle will be just above the knee, where it is to be well secured by many turns of a bandage. The two ends are then to be knotted. If you have no pulleys, a twisted sheet or rope may be passed through the loop formed by the napkin. If you can procure the former, however, cast the loop over the hook of the lower block, and secure the upper one to the wall, directly opposite to hooks or men that hold the sheets that pass between the thighs. A steadily increasing and forcible extension of the thigh is then to be made by men who are stationed at the pulleys or sheet, while you are turning and twisting the limb to assist in dislodging it from its unnatural situation. By these means, properly applied, the head of the bone will frequently slip into its socket with a loud noise.

If, however, you are foiled, change the direction of the extending foice, recollecting always, that it is not by sudden or violent jerk, that any benefit can be attained, but by a steady increasing and long continued pull. Should all your efforts prove unavailing, (I would not advise you to lose much time before you resort to it,) make the patient, as before directed, excessively drunk, and when he cannot stand, apply the pulleys. If this fails, or is objected to, bleed him till he faints, and then try it again.

Dislocation of the Knee-Pan. When this little bone is dislocated, it is evident on the slightest glance. To reduce it, lay the patient on his back, straighten his leg, lift it up to a right angle with his body, and in that position push the bone back to its place. The knee should be kept at rest for a few days.

Dislocation of the Leg. As these accidents cannot happen without tearing and lacerating the soft parts, but little force is required to place the bones in their natural situation. If the paits are so much torn that the bone slips again out of place, apply Hartshorne's or Desaults apparatus for a fractured thigh.

Dislocation of the Foot.—The foot is seldom dislocated. Should it happen, however, let one person secure the leg, and another draw the foot, while you push the bone in the contrary way to that in which it was forced out. The part is then to be covered with compresses dipped in lead water, and a splint applied on each side of the leg, that reaches below the foot. Accidents of this natuie are always dangerous; all that can be done to remedy them, consists in the speedy reduction of the bone, keeping the parts at rest, and subduing the inflammation by following the directions of page 207.

Of Compound Accidents.—Having spoken of the treatment to be pursued for a bruise, wound, fracture, and dislocation, as hapening singly, it remains to state what is to be done when they are united.

We will suppose that a man has been violently thrown from a carriage. On examination a wound is found in his thigh, bleeding profusely; his ankle is out of joint, with a wound communicating with its cavity, and the leg broken.

In the first place, stop the bleeding from the wound in the thigh; reduce the dislocation next; draw the edges of the wounds together with sticking plaster, and lastly, apply Hartshorne's or Dassault's apparatus to the fracture.

If, instead of a wound, fracture, and dislocation, there is a concussion or compression of the brain, a dislocation and fracture, attend to the concussion first, the dislocation next, and the fracture the last.

Of Amputation—As accidents sometimes happen at sea, or in situations where it is impossible to obtain a surgeon, and which require the immediate amputation of a limb, it is proper to say a few words on that subject. To perform the operation is one thing, and to know when it ought to be performed is another. Any man of common dexterity and firmness, can cut off a leg, but to decide upon the necessity of doing so, requires much judgment, instances having occurred where, under the most seemingly desperate circumstances, the patient, through fear or obstinacy, has refusnd to submit to the knife, and yet, afterwards recovered.

Although, in many cases, much doubt may exist in determining whether it is proper to amputate or not, yet, in others, all difficulty vanishes, as when a ball has carried away an arm. Suppose, for a moment, while rolling in a heavy sea, during a gale, the lashings of a gun give way, by which a man has his knee leg or

· ankle completely smashed ; or that either of those parts are crushed by a fall from the top-gallant yard, a falling tree, &c.   The great laceration of blood vessels, nerves and tendons, the crushing and splintering of the bones, almost necessarily resulting from such accidents, render immediate amputation an unavoidable and imperious duty.

If there are none of the regular instruments at hand, you must provide the following, which are always to be bad, and which answer extremely well, being careful to have the knives as sharp and smooth as possible.

Instruments.—The handkerchief and stick, a carving or other large knife with a straight blade, a pen-knife, a carpenter's tenon or mitre saw, a slip of leather or linen, three inches wide and eighteen or twenty long, slit up the middle to the half of its length, a dozen or more ligatures, each about a foot long, made of waxed thread, bobbin, or fine twine, a hook with a sharp point, a pair of slender pincers, several narrow slips of sticking plaster, dry hat, a piece of linen large enough to cover the stump spread with simple ointment or lard, a bandage three or four yards long, the width of your hand, sponges and warm water.

Amputation of the Arm. Operation—Give the patient sixty drops of laudanum, and seat him on a narrow and firm table or chest, of a convenient height, so that some one can support him, by clasping him round the body.   If the handkerchief and stick have not been previously applied, place it as high up the arm as possible, (the stick being very short,) and so that the knot may pass on the inner side of it.   Your instruments having been placed regularly on a table or waiter, and within reach of your hand, while some one supports the lower end of the arm, and at the same time draws down the skin, take the large knife and make one straight cut all round the limb, through the skin and fat only, then with the penknife separate as much of the skin from the flesh above the cut, and all around it, as will form a flap to cover the face of the stump, when you think there is enough separated, turn it back, where it must be held by an assistant, while with the large knife you make a second straight incision round the arm and down to the bone, as close as you can to the double edge of the flap, but taking great care not to cut it. The bone is now to be passed through the slit in the piece of linen before mentioned, and pressed by its ends against the upper surface of the wound by the person who holds the flap, while you saw through the bone as near as you can. With the hooks or pincers, you then seize and tie up every vessel that bleeds, the largest first, and smaller ones next, until they are all secured. When this is done, relax the stick a little; if an artery springs tie it as before. The wound is now to be gently cleansed with a sponge and warm water, and the stick to be relaxed. If it is evident that the arteries are all tied, bring the flap over the stump, draw its edges together with strips of sticking plaster, leaving the ligature hanging out at the angles, lay the piece of linen spread with ointment over the straps, a plaget of linen over that, and secure the whole by the bandage, when the patient may be carried to bed, and the stump laid on a pillow.

The handkerchief and stick are to be left loosely round the limb, so that if any bleeding happens to come on, it may be tightened in an instant by the person who watches by the patient, when the dressings must be taken off, the flap raised, and the vessel be sought for and tied up, after which, every thing is to be placed as before,

It may be well to observe that in sawing through the bone, a long and free stroke should be used to prevent any hitching, as an additional security against which, the teeth of the saw should be well sharpened and set wide.

There is also another circumstance, which it is essen-

tial to be aware of; the ends of divided arteries cannot at times be got hold of, or being diseased their coats
give way under the hook, so that they cannot be drawn
out; sometimes, also, they are found ossified or turned
into bone. In all these cases, having armed a needle
with a ligature, pass it through the flesh round the artery, so that when tied there will be a portion of it included in the ligature along with the artery. When the
ligature has been made to encircle the artery, cut off
the needle, and tie it firmly in the ordinary way.

The bandages, &c., should not be disturbed for five
or six days if the weather is cool; if it is very warm,
they may be removed in three. This is to be done
with the greatest care, soaking them well with warm
water, until they are quite soft, and can be taken away
without sticking to the stump. A clean plaster, lint and
bandage are then to be applied as before, to be removed every two days. At the expiration of fourteen or
fifteen days, the ligatures generally come away; and
in three or four weeks, if every thing goes on well, the
wound heals.

Amputation of the thigh.—This is performed in precisely the same manner as that of the thigh, with one
exception, it being proper to interpose a piece of lint
between the edges of the flap, to prevent them from
uniting, until the face of the stump has adhered to it.

Amputation of the Leg.—As there are two bones in
the leg, which have a thin muscle between, it is necessary to have an additional knife to those already mentioned, to divide it. It should have a long narrow blade,
with a double cutting edge, and a sharp point; a carving
or case knife may be ground down to answer the purpose, the blade being reduced to rather less than half
an inch in width. The linen or leather strip should also
eave two slits in it, instead of one. The patient is to
be laid on his back, on a table covered with blankets or

a mattrass, with a sufficient number of assistants to secure him.   The handkerchief and stick being applied
on the upper part of the thigh, one person holds the
knee and another the foot and leg, as steadily as possi.
ble, while, with the large knife, the operator makes an
oblique incision around the limb, through the skin, and
beginning at five or six inches below the knee-pan, and
carrying it regularly around in such manner that the
cut will be lower down on the calf than in front of
the leg.   As much of the skin is then to be separated
by the penknife, as will cover the stump.   When this
is turned back, a second cut is to be made all round
the limb and down to the bones, when, with the narrow bladed knife, just mentioned, the flesh between
them is to be divided.   The middle piece of the leather
strip is now to be pulled through between the bones,
the whole being held back by the assistant, who supports the flaps while the bones are sawed, which should
be so managed that the smaller one is completely cut
through by the time the other is half so.   The arteries
are then to be taken up, the flap brought down and
secured by adhesive plaster, &c., as already directed.

Amputation of the Fore-Arm—As the fore-arm has
two bones in it, the narrow bladed knife, and the strip of
linen with three tails, are to be provided.   The incision
should be straight around the part, as in the arm, with
this exception, complete it as directed for the preceding
case.

Amputation of Fingers and Toes—Draw the skin
back, and make an incision round the finger, a little below the joint it is intended to remove, turn back a little
flap to cover the stump, then cut down to the joint, bending it so that you can cut through the ligaments that
connect the two bones, the under one first, then that
on the side.   The head of the bone is then to be turn-

17

ed out, while you cut through the remaining soft part If you see any artery spirt, tie it up—if not, bring down the flap and secure it by a strip of sticking plaster, and a narrow bandage over the whole.

Remarks.—To prevent the troublesome consequences of secondary bleeding,before the strips of plaster are applied over the edges of the flap, give the patient, if he is faint, a little wine and water, and wait a few minutes to see whether the increased force it gives to the circulation, will occasion a flow of blood, if it does, secure the vessel it comes from. If there is a considerable flow of blood from the hollow of the bone, place a small cedar plug in it. Should violent spasms of the stump ensue, have it carefully held by assistants, and give the patient large doses of laudanum; it may, in fact, be laid down as a general rule, that after every operation of this kind, laudanum should be given in greater or less doses, as the patient may be in more or less pain.

NATURAL PHILOSOPHY.

We may admire that a varied edifice, or even a magnificent city, can be constructed of stone from one quarry; yet, far surpassing this, it is found that the inconceivably, more varied and magnificent fabric of the universe, with all its orders of phenomena, is of elements but a little more complex.

The four words, *Atom, Attraction, Repulsion,* and *Stubborness,* the reader's eye may be fixed on, as four physical parts of nature, while we treat on them.

1st. *Atom*—from the Greek word signifying that which cannot be further divided. The earth, as well as other bodies, are made up of such particles, and held together by attraction.

2nd. *Attraction* — is that which draws substances to. gether.

3rd. *Repulsion* — is that which operates against at. traction, and throws substances apart, as when heated water bursts into steam, or gunpowder explodes.

4th. *Inertia* — expresses the fact, that the atoms, in regard to motion, have about them what may be figu. ratively called a state — whatever it may be — in other words, that bodies neither acquire motion, nor lose motion, nor bend their course in motion, but in exact proportion to some force applied.

It is worthy of notice, that in learning any thing, the scholar's eye should be fixed on all the connecting parts, and comprehend them in as small bounds as possible, so as to give a general view of the whole — as when a person is learning geography they should have a map of the whole world immediately before them, and as they examine any country they can connect it with the rest, having their courses and climates.

The universe is built of very minute or small atoms, called matter, which by mutual attraction cling together in masses of various forms and sizes. The smallest substance which the human eye can see is still a mass of many atoms of matter, which may be separated from each other, or arranged differently; still they cannot be destroyed or annihilated.

A small mass of gold may be hammered into thin leaf, or drawn into fine wire, or cut into almost invisible parts, or liquified in a crucible, or dissolved in acid, or dissipated by intense heat into vapors, yet after any and all of these changes, the atoms can be collected again to form the original gold, without the slightest diminution. And all the substances or elements of which our globe is composed, may thus be cut, torn, bruised, ground, &c. a thousand times, but are always recoverable as perfect as at first.

And with respect to delicate combinations of these elements, such as exist in animal and vegetable substances, although it be beyond human art originally to produce or even closely to imitate many of them, still in their decomposition and apparent destruction, the accomplished chemist of the present day does not lose a single atom. The coal which burns in his apparatus, until only a little ashes remain behind, or the wax taper which seems to vanish altogether in flame, or the portion of animal flesh which putrifies, and gradually dries up and disappears — present to us phenomena which are now proved to be only changes of connection and arrangement, among the indestructible ultimate atoms, and the chemist can offer all the elements again mixed or separate, as desired, for any of the useful purposes to which they are severally applicable.

A grain of blue vitriol, or carmine, will tinge a gallon of water so that in every drop the color may be perceived.

The buzzard smells his food at a considerable distance, and that is done by small atoms flying in the air.

Any substance when sufficiently heated, rises as invisible vapor. Great heat, therefore, would cause the whole of the material universe to disappear, the most solid bodies becoming as invisible as the air we breathe in.

Mutual Attraction. — The earth, though it is made up of many different materials and elements, according to a geographical description, is said to be round; the sun, moon, and stars, or heavenly bodies, are also round, as well as the thousand instances of melted metal that gather into round substances, like the lead allowed to rain down from an elevated seive, which, by cooling as it descends, retains the form of liquid drops, and becomes the shot lead to shoot with; as well as the rain drops, dew drops, and drops of mercury, gather in round substances.

Thus a plummet suspended near the side of a mountain, is drawn toward it in a degree proportioned to the size of the mountain by the side of the earth, and the reason why the plummet tends more towards the earth than the mountain, is because the earth is larger than the mountain.

Logs of wood, floating in water, approach each other, and afterwards generally remain together. The wreck of a ship, in a smooth sea, after a storm is often seen gathered into heaps. These things show the power of attraction.

The cause of the extraordinary phenomenon which we call attraction, acts at all distances. The moon, though two hundred and forty thousand miles from the earth, by her attraction raises the water of the ocean under her, and forms what we call the tide. The sun, still further off, has similar influences, and when the sun and moon act in the same direction, we have the spring tides. The plannets are so far distant that they appear to us little wandering points in the heavens, yet by their attraction effect the motion of our earth in her orbit, quickening it when she is approaching them, and retarding it when she is receding.

The attraction is greater the nearer the bodies are to each other, and less as they get off farther. Like the light of a candle, that close by appears very evident, but grows dimmer as we get further off. Thus, a board an inch square, one foot from a light, Just covers a board of two inches, two feet off, and so increases as we get further off; and as the light spreads over more surface it grows weaker, in proportion to the surface that it covers. Light and attraction act alike in this sense. What weighs 1000 pounds at the sea shore, weighs five pounds less at the top of a mountain of a certain height, or raised in a balloon—as is proved experimentally by a spring ballance—and at the distance of the moon the weight or force toward the earth of 1000 pounds is diminished to five ounces, as is proved by astronomical tests.

Attraction has received different names as it is found

acting under different circumstances. The chief distinctions are gravitation, cohesion, capillary and chemical attraction.

Gravitation is the name given to it when it acts at a great distance. Cohesion is the name given when it acts at a very short distance, as in keeping the atoms of a mass together. Attraction is called capillary when it acts between a liquid and a solid, which has tubes or pores—attraction has received the name of Chemical attraction when it unites the atoms of two or more distinct substances into one perfect compound.

Dr. Arnott says—It might appear at first sight that it cannot be the same cause which draws a piece of iron to the earth with the moderate force, called its weight, and which maintains the constituent atoms of the iron in such strong cohesion; but when we recollect that attraction is stronger as the substances are nearer to each other, the difficulty vanishes. Atoms, in absolute contact, would be a million times, nay, infinitely nearer to each other, than when only a quarter of an inch apart; and, therefore, when the heat among the atoms of any cohering mass allows them to approach near, they must attract mutually with great force.

I would not offer to contradict the doctor in these last remarks, yet I possess some small doubts whether every thing that is stated in this last point is correct.— One is, whether the word *infinite* would apply in that place; and another is, whether it is not the kind of metal that maintains the strength as well as atoms, being close together, though he might argue that this was the reason why it was stronger, that the atoms were closer than other metal—though he has brought forward many more evidences, that I have not room in this piece to quote.

Were it not, then, because the surfaces of bodies are in general so very rough and irregular, that if applied to each other they can only touch. perhaps, in four or five points out of a million, which the surface contains bodies would invariably stick together, or cohering by any accidental contact, the effect of artificially smoothing the touching surfaces, is seen in the following ex. amples.

Similar portions being cut off with a clean knife from two leaden bullets, and the fresh surfaces being bro't into contact with a light turning pressure, the bullets cohere almost as it they had been originally cast together.

Two small, of perfectly smooth plates of glass or marble, laid upon each other, adhere with great force; and, indeed, so do most well polished flat surfaces.

Repulsion is often effected by heat. Were there only atoms and attraction, as has been explained, the whole material of creation would rush into close contact, forming one huge solid mass of stillness and death. But there is also heat which counteracts attraction.— When a continued addition of heat is made to any substance, it gradually increases the mutual distance of the constituent atoms. or dilates the body a solid; thus it is first softened, then melted, or fused, that is to say, reduced to the state of liquid, as the cohesive attraction is overcome. And lastly, the atoms are repelled to still greater distances, so that the substance is converted into elastic fluid or air. Abstraction of heat from such air, causes a return of states into the reverse order. Ice, when heated, thus becomes water, and the water when heated further becomes steam, when cooled again becomes water as before, and the water becomes ice. Other substances are similarly affected by heat; but as all have different relations to it, some requiring much more heat for liquifaction, and some very little. We therefore have that beautiful variety of solids, liquids. and air, which makes up our external nature. For instance, a rod of iron which, when cold, will pass through a certain opening, and will lie lengthwise between two fixed points; but when heated, becomes too thick and too long to do either. The common ther-

mometer for measuring the degrees of heat, is a glas-
filled with mercury, or other fluid, and having a nars
row tube rising from it, into which the fluid ascends on
being expanded by heat, and so makes the degree.

A bladder of cold air, on being heated, becomes
tight, and in certain cases will burst.

As different materials require a different degree of
heat to dissolve them, so gold requires 5000 degrees,
lead 600, ice 32, &c., and if heating be afterwards continued, most things at certain higher temperatures suddenly expand again to many times the present size, until the liquid becomes airiform fluid. · One pint of water, driven off as steam from the boiler of a low pressure steam engine, fills a space of nearly 2000 pints.
On the earth, near the equator, common sealing wax
will not retain impressions, but is oil in the day, and a
soft solid at night; and tallow candles cannot be used;
and near our pole in winter the water is hard, and so
are the different oils; thus we see that heat causes repulsion, as well as wind, water or fire, when pressed,
will explode, as well as gunpowder. These are the
most common means of repulsion.

Were there no motion in the universe, it would be
dead—it would be without the rising or setting sun—
or rivers flowing—or circulation of wind—and there
would be neither sounds nor light, or animal existence.
Motion is only understood by comparing one object
with others, and perhaps the other objects are in motion at the same time. This earth is thought to have
three motions when compared with the heavenly bodies. One is the motion of a circuit round the sun eve-
ery year; another is rolling over every twenty-four
hours; and the third is rocking toward the sun and
from it once a year.

Life and motion are closely connected. The blood,
which is the life, is in a perpetual motion as long as
life is known in man or beast, and even in fish, fowl
or insects. I ask, where do we find life without mo-

tion?' We may say, no where. Then, where does the argument arise, that people must not stir nor exer_cise, or they will bring on the disease again? We may say, not from the laws of life, but rather from the laws of death. Then, according to the laws that have been explained, if attraction draws substances together, this agrees with that part of the system that humors, flocking together, and settling together in the body, and also, that the matter or gluten of the blood gather into bodies, and thus checks the organs or blood vessels. If that law, called Repulsion, disperses bodies (and it is mostly effected by beat,)as is believed, according to the laws of nature, this agrees with the system which states that heat drives diseases, as well as those thick substances which are in the blood ; therefore it ought to be applied to the whole body, but more particularly to the inside—that is, by steam, which goes to the heart and lights, and hot teas on the stomach. This will drive diseases out towards the surface of the body.

Law of Inertia—That bodies tend to continue in the state of motion, or of rest, in which they happen to be, so to render force necessary to change the state, is seen in the following facts. The scientific term uesd to express this law is *Inertia*—but sometimes the *obstinacy* and *stubbornness* have been substituted. for explanation. When the sails of a ship are first spread to receive the force of the wind, the vessels does not get in full speed at once, but slowly, as the continued force gradually overcomes the inertia of her mass. If the sails are, after she gets in speed, suddenly taken down, she does not lose her speed at once, but slowly again, as the continued resisting force of the water destroys it, Horses must make a greater effort at first to put a carriage into motion than to maintain the motion afterwards, and a strong, effort is required to stop a moving carriage. When a carriage body, hanging with springs, first begins to move, the body of it appears to fall back, and a person within seems to be suddenly thrown against the back cushion. When the carriage stops again the body swings forward. A bad rider on horse-back may be left behind when his horse darts off suddenly, or may be thrown off on one side by the horse starting to the other. A horse at speed stopping suddenly, often sends his rider over his head. A man setting in a ship cabin, where the air that is on the outside has no communication, through the ship may move forward ten miles an hour, he scarcely knows whether it is going forward or backward, or at rest. If he throws up a ball it will fall back, just as if he was on the land. This shows that the ball has relative motion with the ship—and though the man may have all the furniture with him that he could wish, he cannot discover from any thing inside of the cabin that the ship is moving. Thus we may be enclosed inside of this atmosphere, while the earth moves as rapidly as it is said to do, and we be insenible of it.— Many more circumstances might he numerated ; but these may suffice to show the law of stubborness.

The author takes the liberty to state, that in addition to the means that have been laid down for the cure of the consumption, he has applied large plasters of No. 6, on the back of a number of persons, and when they have sweat so free that the plasters have slipped off, he has renewed them till the patient got well ; and in the course of the last year there has been about 25 professed to be cured of the above disease.

I have observed that among those persons who have purchased my rights there are some of almost every order ; some medical men, some Thompsonians, Indian doctors, (so called) Water doctors, Botanical, &c. as well as a considerable number that never have been doctors at all ; each possessing, in a greater or less degree, their habitual prejudices ; yet there has been almost universal harmony and friendship among them, though many of them differ widely in their religious and political sentiments. The philanthropic spirit has prepailed to a great extent. But those who have kept nearest the system have generally had the best luck. Some have given the emetic in warm weak lie, instead of cold, and then complained of its not operating right. But I have not heard of many complaint where it has been given right, tho' we should use the second species. And I have not heard of any changes for the better. Here I notice, that when No. 4 is used for cleansing the blood, or enlivening the bowels by repeated portions at any time, let it be of the second species; but if it is given for worms, let it be of the first species.

As this system will likely be deterred by some of the state laws which are unconstitutional, I will remark, that in contending with them, we should always refer to the constitution of the State, or the United States. One point is, that there shall be no law made that shall destroy the validity of many contract. Another that there shall be no law made that a person shall have something for nothing. These are common points; and every officer, when sworn into office, is bound to support the Constitution of the United States. And one point in the Constitution is, to grant patents. Hence they are to support the Patent Law, but they are not bound to support unconstitutional laws.

The general means for cures or common processes, as are laid down in the book, has been applied to women for the rise and obstruction of the menses to advantage, and they have been applied in almost every stage of pregnancy without danger.

MATERIA MEDICA.

SURGERY.

Lightning Source UK Ltd.
Milton Keynes UK
UKHW02f2021270818
327886UK00014B/1238/P